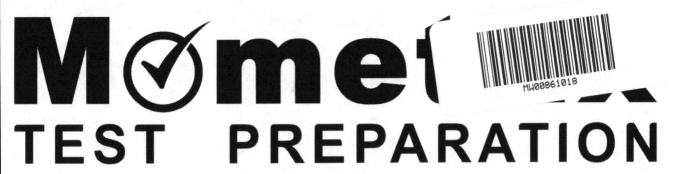

TEST PREPARATION

Nursing Acceleration Challenge Exam (ACE) I PN-RN: Foundations of Nursing Secrets Study Guide Part 2 of 2

DEAR FUTURE EXAM SUCCESS STORY

First of all, **THANK YOU** for purchasing Mometrix study materials!

Second, congratulations! You are one of the few determined test-takers who are committed to doing whatever it takes to excel on your exam. **You have come to the right place.** We developed these study materials with one goal in mind: to deliver you the information you need in a format that's concise and easy to use.

In addition to optimizing your guide for the content of the test, we've outlined our recommended steps for breaking down the preparation process into small, attainable goals so you can make sure you stay on track.

We've also analyzed the entire test-taking process, identifying the most common pitfalls and showing how you can overcome them and be ready for any curveball the test throws you.

Standardized testing is one of the biggest obstacles on your road to success, which only increases the importance of doing well in the high-pressure, high-stakes environment of test day. Your results on this test could have a significant impact on your future, and this guide provides the information and practical advice to help you achieve your full potential on test day.

Your success is our success

We would love to hear from you! If you would like to share the story of your exam success or if you have any questions or comments in regard to our products, please contact us at **800-673-8175** or **support@mometrix.com**.

Thanks again for your business and we wish you continued success!

Sincerely,
The Mometrix Test Preparation Team

> **Need more help? Check out our flashcards at:**
> **http://MometrixFlashcards.com/NursingACE**

TABLE OF CONTENTS

Psychosocial

Sexual Orientation

SEXUALITY

Sexuality is an integral part of each individual's personality and refers to all aspects of being a sexual human. It is more than just the act of physical intercourse. A person's sexuality is often apparent in what they do, in their appearance, and in how they interact with others. There are four main aspects of sexuality:

- **Genetic identity** or chromosomal gender
- **Gender identification** or how they perceive themselves with regard to male or female
- **Gender role** or the attributes of their cultural role
- **Sexual orientation** or the gender to which one is attracted

By assessing and attempting to conceptualize a person's sexuality, the social worker can gain a broader understanding of the client's beliefs and will be able to provide a more holistic approach to providing care.

GENDER IDENTITY

Gender identity is the gender to which the individual identifies, which may or may not be the gender of birth (natal gender). Most children begin to express identification and behaviors associated with gender between ages 2 and 4. The degree to which this identification is influenced by genetics and environment is an ongoing debate because, for example, female children are often socialized toward female roles (dresses, dolls, pink items). Societal pressure to conform to gender stereotypes is strong, so gender dysphoria, which is less common in early childhood than later, may be suppressed. At the onset of puberty, sexual attraction may further complicate gender identity although those with gender dysphoria most often have sexual attraction to those of the same natal gender, so a natal boy who identifies as a girl is more likely to be sexually attracted to boys than to girls. Later in adolescence, individuals generally experiment with sexual behavior and solidify their gender identity.

INFLUENCE OF SEXUAL ORIENTATION ON BEHAVIORS

The degree to which sexual orientation influences behavior may vary widely depending on the individual. For example, some gay males may be indistinguishable in appearance and general behavior from heterosexual males while others may behave in a stereotypically flamboyant manner. The same holds true for lesbians, with some typically feminine in appearance and behavior and others preferring a more masculine appearance. The typical heterosexual model (two people in a stable relationship) is increasingly practiced by homosexual couples while others prefer less traditional practices. Depending on the degree of acceptance that LGBTQ individuals encounter, they may hide their sexual orientation or maintain a heterosexual relationship in order to appear straight. LGBTQ individuals are at higher risk of depression and suicide, especially if they experience rejection because of their sexual orientation or have been taught that it is sinful. LGBTQ individuals with multiple sexual partners (especially males) are at increased risk for STDs, including HIV/AIDS.

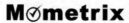

COMING OUT PROCESS

The coming out process is the act of revealing LGBTQ sexual orientation to family and friends. This generally occurs during adolescence or early adulthood although some may delay coming out for decades or never do so. Individuals may come out to select groups of people. For example, friends may be aware of an individual's orientation but not family or co-workers. Coming out can be frightening for many people, especially if they have reason to fear rejection or fear for their safety. Stages in coming out typically progress in the following order:

Stage	Actions and feelings involved
Confusion	The individual may be unsure of feelings or be in denial.
Exploration	The individual begins to question orientation and wonder about LGBTQ people.
Breakthrough	The individual accepts the likelihood of being LGBTQ and seeks others of the same orientation.
Acceptance	The individual accepts orientation and begins to explore and read about the LGBTQ culture.
Pride	The individual begins to exhibit pride in orientation and may reject straight culture or exhibit stereotypically LGBTQ behaviors.
Synthesis	The individual comes to terms with the reality of the LGBTQ orientation, is at peace with their identity, and is generally out to family, friends, and co-workers.

PRACTICE ISSUES WHEN WORKING WITH LGBTQ CLIENTS

Possible practice issues with LGBTQ clients include, but are not limited to, the following:

- Stigmatization and violence
- Internalized homophobia
- Coming out
- AIDS
- Limited civil rights
- Orientation vs. preference (biology vs. choice)

Problematic treatment models for treating gay and lesbian people include the following:

- The moral model for treatment is religiously oriented and views homosexuality as sinful.
- Reparative or conversion psychotherapy focuses on changing a person's sexual orientation to heterosexual. Traditional mental health disciplines view this type of treatment as unethical and as having no empirical base.

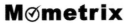

Self-Image

FACTORS INFLUENCING SELF-IMAGE

Factors influencing self-image include the following:

- **Spirituality**: Religious or spiritual beliefs may affect how individuals see their place in the world and their self-confidence. Individuals may gain self-esteem through secure beliefs and membership in a like group, but belief systems with a strong emphasis on sin may impair self-image.
- **Culture**: Individuals are affected (negatively and positively) by cultural expectations, especially if they feel outside of the norm.
- **Ethnicity**: Whether or not the individual is part of the dominant ethnic group may have a profound effect on self-image. Minority groups often suffer discrimination that reinforces the idea that they are less valuable than others.
- **Education**: Those with higher levels of education tend to have a better self-image than those without, sometimes because of greater unemployment and fewer opportunities associated with low education.
- **Gender**: Society often reinforces the value of males (straight) over females and LGBTQ individuals.
- **Abuse**: Those who are abused may often develop a poor self-image, believing they are deserving of abuse.
- **Media**: The media reinforces stereotypes and presents unrealistic (and unattainable) images, affecting self-image.

BODY IMAGE

Body image is the perception individuals have of their own bodies, positive or negative. An altered body image may result in a number of responses, most often beginning during adolescence but sometimes during childhood:

- **Obesity**: Some may be unhappy with their body image and overeat as a response, often increasing their discontent.
- **Eating disorders**: Some may react to being overweight or to the cultural ideal by developing anorexia or bulimia in an attempt to achieve the idealized body image they seek. They may persist even though they put their lives at risk. Their body image may be so distorted that they believe they are fat even when emaciated.
- **Body dysmorphic disorder**: Some may develop a preoccupation with perceived defects in their body image, such as a nose that is too big or breasts or penis that is too small. Individuals may become obsessed to the point that they avoid social contact with others, stop participating in sports, get poor grades, stop working, or seek repeated plastic surgery.

Grief and Loss

GRIEF

Grief is an emotional response to a **loss** that begins at the time a loss is anticipated and continues on an individual timetable. While there are identifiable stages or tasks, it is not an orderly and predictable process. It involves overcoming anger, disbelief, guilt, and a myriad of related emotions. The grieving individual may move back and forth between stages or experience several emotions at any given time. Each person's grief response is unique to their own coping patterns, stress levels, age, gender, belief system, and previous experiences with loss.

KUBLER-ROSS'S FIVE STAGES OF GRIEF

Kubler-Ross taught the medical and nursing community that the dying patient and family welcomes open, honest discussion of the dying process and felt that there were certain **stages** that patients and family go through. The stages may not occur in order, but may vary or some may be skipped. Stages include:

- **Denial**: The person denies the diagnosis and tries to pretend it isn't true. During this time, the person may seek a second opinion or alternative therapies. They may use denial until they are better able to emotionally cope with the reality of the disease or changes that need to be made. Patients may also wish to save family and friends from pain and worry. Both patients and family may use denial as a coping mechanism when they feel overwhelmed by the reality of the disease and threatened losses.
- **Anger**: The person is angry about the situation and may focus that rage on anyone.
- **Bargaining**: The person attempts to make deals with a higher power to secure a better outcome to their situation.
- **Depression**: The person anticipates the loss and the changes it will bring with a sense of sadness and grief.
- **Acceptance**: The person accepts the impending death and is ready to face it as it approaches. The patient may begin to withdraw from interests and family.

> **Review Video: Patient Treatment and Grief**
> Visit mometrix.com/academy and enter code: 648794

ANTICIPATORY GRIEF

Anticipatory grief is the mental, social, and somatic reactions of an individual as they prepare themselves for a **perceived future loss**. The individual experiences a process of intellectual, emotional, and behavioral responses in order to modify their self-concept, based on their perception of what the potential loss will mean in their life. This process often takes place ahead of the actual loss, from the time the loss is first perceived until it is resolved as a reality for the individual. This process can also blend with past loss experiences. It is associated with the individual's perception of how life will be affected by the particular diagnosis as well as the impending death. Acknowledging this anticipatory grief allows family members to begin looking toward a changed future. Suppressing this anticipatory process may inhibit relationships with the ill individual and contribute to a more difficult grieving process at a later time. However, appropriate anticipatory grieving does not take the place of grief during the actual time of death.

DISENFRANCHISED GRIEF

Disenfranchised grief occurs when the loss being experienced cannot be openly acknowledged, publicly mourned, or socially supported. Society and culture are partly responsible for an individual's response to a loss. There is a **social context** to grief; if a person incurring the loss will be putting himself or herself at risk if grief is expressed, disenfranchised grief occurs. The risk for disenfranchised grief is greatest among those whose relationship with the individual they lost was not known or regarded as significant. This is also the situation found among bereaved persons who are not recognized by society as capable of grief, such as young children, or needing to mourn, such as an ex-spouse or secret lover.

GRIEF VS. DEPRESSION

Normal grief is preoccupied with self-limiting to the loss itself. Emotional responses will vary and may include open expressions of anger. The individual may experience difficulty sleeping or vivid dreams, a lack of energy, and weight loss. Crying is evident and provides some relief of extreme emotions. The individual remains socially responsive and seeks reassurance from others.

Depression is marked by extensive periods of sadness and preoccupation often extending beyond 2 months. It is not limited to the single event. There is an absence of pleasure or anger and isolation from previous social support systems. The individual can experience extreme lethargy, weight loss, insomnia, or hypersomnia, and has no recollection of dreaming. Crying is absent or persistent and provides no relief of emotions. Professional intervention is required to relieve depression.

LOSS

Loss is the blanket term used to denote the absence of a valued object, position, ability, attribute, or individual. The aspect of **loss** as it is associated with the death of an animal or person is a relatively new definition. Loss is an individualized and subjective experience depending on the **perceived attachment** between the individual and the missing aspect. This can range from little or no value of attachment to significant value. Loss also can be represented by the **withdrawal of a valued relationship** one had or would have had in the future. Depending on the unique and individual responses to the perception of loss and its significance, reactions to the loss will vary. Robinson and McKenna summarize the aspects of loss in three main attributes:

- Something has been removed.
- The item removed had value to that person.
- The response is individualized.

MOURNING

Mourning is a public grief response for the death of a loved one. The various aspects of the mourning process are partially determined by **personal and cultural belief systems**. Kagawa-Singer defines mourning as "the social customs and cultural practices that follow a death." Durkheim expands this to include the following: "mourning is not a natural movement of private feelings wounded by a cruel loss; it is a duty imposed by the group." Mourning involves participation in religious and culturally appropriate customs and rituals designed to publicly acknowledge the loss. These rituals signify they are adjusting to the change in their relationships created by the loss, as well as mark the beginning of the reorganization and forward movement of their lives.

BEREAVEMENT

Bereavement is the emotional and mental state associated with having suffered a **personal loss**. It is the reactions of grief and sadness initiated by the loss of a loved one. Bereavement is a normal process of feeling deprived of something of value. The word bereave comes from the root "reave" meaning to plunder, spoil, or rob. It is recognized that the lost individual had value and a defining role in the surviving individual's life. Bereavement encompasses all the acts and emotions surrounding the feeling of loss for the individual. During this grieving period, there is an increased mortality risk. A **positive bereavement experience** means being able to recognize the significance of the loss while still recognizing the resilience and value of life.

RISK FACTORS COMPLICATING BEREAVEMENT

The caregiver should assess for multiple **life crises** that take energy away from the grieving process. An important factor is the grieving individual's history with past grieving experiences. Assess for other recent, unresolved, or difficult losses that may need to be addressed before the individual can move toward resolution of the current loss. Age, mental health, substance abuse, extreme anger, anxiety, or dependence on the individual facing the end of life can add additional stressors and handicap natural coping mechanisms. Income strains, community support, outside and personal responsibilities, the absence of cultural and religious beliefs, the difficulty of the disease process, and age of the loved one lost can also present additional risk factors.

COUNSELING AND PROVIDING EMOTIONAL SUPPORT REGARDING GRIEF AND LOSS TO CHILDREN

The approach to counseling and providing emotional support regarding grief and loss to children is dependent on the age of the child. When available, children and family should be provided information about **peer support groups** (especially adolescents) and **bereavement art therapy groups** as these may be especially helpful. The nurse should use appropriate words (death, died) instead of euphemisms (went to sleep) when talking about the deceased and should encourage the child to ask questions. Children are often reluctant to express feelings directly, so it may be beneficial to encourage them to keep a journal about their feelings or draw pictures to express them. Parents should be encouraged to share their feelings of grief with their children rather than trying to hide their emotions and should be aware that children express grief in different ways and may regress or complain of physical ailments (stomach ache, headache) in response to grief. Children should be prepared for changes in routines or living situations, such as a stay-at-home parent having to take a job, which may occur as a result of a death or serious illness.

SIGNS OF A CHILD HAVING ISSUES MANAGING GRIEF

Management of **grief** comes in stages for children as well as for adults. Grief may be complicated for a child who does not understand the significance of the situation, such as in the case of a parent's death, or for someone who does not have the necessary support systems in place, as in the case of a child who has a grieving parent who consequently becomes unavailable. **Signs that a child is not coping well with grief** include extended periods of sadness, lack of interest in regular activities, sleep disturbances, loss of appetite, statements of wishing for death or joining a person who has died, difficulties with concentration, problems taking direction at school, poor school performance, and fear of being alone.

NURSING INTERVENTIONS FOR PATIENTS AND FAMILY EXPERIENCING LOSS AND GRIEF

Loss is painful and frightening. Loss can occur through death or loss of health, self-esteem, or relationships. Loss can also occur from threats, such as fire, flood, theft, or severe weather. The severity of the loss, preparation for it, and the maturity, stability, and coping mechanisms of the person all affect the grieving process. Multiple losses and substance abuse can complicate grief and recovery. Previous life experience and cultural and religious beliefs can help in resolution of grief. Many emotions are triggered, and if the loss is not acknowledged, the person may become depressed or develop health problems. **Nursing interventions** for those experiencing **loss and grief** include:

- Teach patients to recognize symptoms, such as SOB, empty feelings in the chest or abdomen, deep sighing, lethargy, and weakness as signs of grief.
- Assist the patient and family to heal themselves by accepting the loss, recognizing the pain from it, making changes to adapt to and assimilate the loss, and moving toward new relationships and activity.
- Refer to groups or counseling for more intense support if needed.

SUPPORTING FAMILIES AND PATIENTS AS THEY RECEIVE BAD NEWS

It is best if the patient and family can **receive bad news** while being **supported** by a team that includes physicians, nurses, and social workers or clergy of their choice. However, the patient may not want family members or others to be present, and this should be respected.

- Provide privacy and ensure that there will be no interruptions.
- Provide seating for all participants.
- Do not provide too much information at once, as the opening statement may be all that the patient can comprehend at one time.
- Allow time for reactions before providing more information.
- Wait for the patient to signal the need for more information and then provide an honest answer in layman's terms. Information may not be absorbed and may need to be repeated as the patient and family are ready for it later after the initial conference.
- Use techniques of therapeutic communication. People may need others to sit and listen and provide comforting empathy many times before having a conversation about problem solving.

SPIRITUALITY

Spirituality provides a connection of the self to a higher power and a way of finding meaning in life experiences. It provides guidance for behavior and can help to clarify one's purpose in life. It can offer hope to those who are ill or facing loss and grief and can give comfort, support, and guidance. **Spirituality** is not always connected to a religion and is highly individualized. A person may lose faith and confidence in his/her spiritual beliefs during trying times:

- Ask patients about their spiritual beliefs.
- Listen attentively and do not offer opinions about their beliefs or share your own unless invited.
- Show respect for their views and offer to obtain spiritual support by calling a spiritual leader or setting up a spiritual ritual that has meaning for them.

This support can help them to regain their beliefs and endure illness by helping them to rise above their suffering and find meaning in this experience.

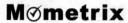

PALLIATIVE AND HOSPICE CARE

Palliative care attempts to make the rest of the patient's life as comfortable as possible by treating distressing symptoms to keep them controlled. It does not attempt to cure but only to control discomfort caused by the disease. Palliative care does not require terminal illness/prognosis and can be implemented for any patient with chronic disease and suffering.

Hospice care uses palliative care as it supports the patient and family through the dying process. Hospice teams support the daily needs of the patient and family and provide needed equipment, medical expertise, and medications to control symptoms. They offer spiritual, psychological, and social support to the patient and family as needed and desired. Assistance with end-of-life planning is given to help the patient and family accomplish goals important to them. Bereavement support is also given. The team consists of the attending physician, hospice physician advisor, nurses, social worker, clergy, hospice aides, and volunteers. Hospice care is given in the home when the patient has family who are willing to assume care with the assistance of the hospice team. Hospice care also occurs in hospice facilities, hospitals, and extended care facilities. To qualify for Hospice care, the patient must be deemed terminal and given a 6-month or less life expectancy by two separate physicians. Should the patient survive 6 months in hospice, they can be extended for two 90-day periods, and then an unlimited number of 60-day periods per physician order.

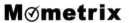

Abuse and Neglect

INDICATORS OF ABUSE THAT MAY BE IDENTIFIED IN THE PATIENT HISTORY

The nurse should always be aware of the presence of any **indicators** that may present a potential for or an actual situation that involves **abuse**. These indicators may present in the **patient's history**. Some examples of indicators concerning their primary complaint may include the following: vague description about the cause of the problem, inconsistencies between physical findings and explanations, minimizing injuries, long period of time between injury and treatment, and over-reactions or under-reactions of family members to injuries. Other important information may be revealed in the family genome, such as family history of violence, time spent in jail or prison, and family history of violent deaths or substance abuse. The patient's health history may include previous injuries, spontaneous abortions, or history of pervious inpatient psychiatric treatment or substance abuse.

During the collection of the patient history, the financial history, the patient's family values, and the patient's relationships with family members can also reveal actual or potential **abuse indicators**.

- The **financial history** may indicate that the patient has little or no money or that they are not given access to money by a controlling family member. They may also be unemployed or utilizing an elderly family member's income for their own personal expenses.
- **Family values** may indicate strong beliefs in physical punishment, dictatorship within the home, inability to allow different opinions within the home, or lack of trust for anyone outside the family.
- **Relationships** within the family may be dysfunctional. Problems such as lack of affection between family members, co-dependency, frequent arguments, extramarital affairs, or extremely rigid beliefs about roles within the family may be present.

During the collection of the patient history, the sexual, social, and psychological history of the patient should be evaluated for any signs of actual or potential abuse.

- The **sexual history** may reveal problems such as previous sexual abuse, forced sexual acts, sexually transmitted diseases, sexual knowledge beyond normal age-appropriate knowledge, or promiscuity.
- The **social history** may reveal unplanned pregnancies, social isolation as evidenced by lack of friends available to help the patient, unreasonable jealousy of significant other, verbal aggression, belief in physical punishment, or problems in school.
- During the **psychological assessment** the patient may express feelings of helplessness and being trapped. The patient may be unable to describe their future, become tearful, perform self-mutilation, have low self-esteem, and have had previous suicide attempts.

NURSING OBSERVATIONS THAT MAY INDICATE ABUSE

During the nursing assessment, observations may also be made by the nurse that can provide vital information about actual or potential abuse. **General observations** may include finding that the patient history is far different from what is objectively viewed by the nurse or that there is a lack of proper clothing or lack of physical care provided. The home environment may include lack of heat, water, or food. It may also reveal inappropriate sleeping arrangements or lack of an environmentally safe housing situation. Observations concerning **family communications** may reveal that the abuser answers all the questions for the whole family or that others look to the controlling member for approval or seem fearful of others. Family members may frequently argue, interrupt each other, or act out negative nonverbal behaviors while others are speaking. They may avoid talking about certain subjects that they feel are secretive.

INDICATORS OF ABUSE THAT MAY BE EVIDENT DURING THE PHYSICAL ASSESSMENT

During the **physical assessment** the nurse should always be aware of any **indicators of abuse**. These indicators may include increased anxiety about being examined or in the presence of the abuser; poor hygiene; looks to abuser to answer questions for them; flinching; over or underweight; presence of bruises, welts, scars or cigarette burns; bald patches on scalp for pulling out of hair; intracranial bleeding; subconjunctival hemorrhages; black eye(s); hearing loss from untreated infection or injury; poor dental hygiene; abdominal injuries; fractures; developmental delays; hyperactive reflexes; genital lacerations or ecchymosis; and presence of sexually transmitted diseases, rectal bruising, bleeding, edema, or poor sphincter tone.

IDENTIFYING AND REPORTING NEGLECT OR LACK OF SUPERVISION IN CHILDREN

While some children may not be physically or sexually abused, they may suffer from profound **neglect** or **lack of supervision** that places them at risk. Indicators include the following:

- Appearing dirty and unkempt, sometimes with infestations of lice, and wearing ill-fitting or torn clothes and shoes
- Being tired and sleepy during the daytime
- Having untended medical or dental problems, such as dental caries
- Missing appointments and not receiving proper immunizations
- Being underweight for stage of development

Neglect can be difficult to assess, especially if the nurse is serving a homeless or very poor population. Home visits may be needed to ascertain if adequate food, clothing, or supervision is being provided; this may be beyond the care provided by the nurse, so suspicions should be reported to appropriate authorities, such as child protective services, so that social workers can assess the home environment.

IDENTIFYING AND REPORTING NEGLECT OF THE BASIC NEEDS OF ADULTS

Neglect of the basic needs of adults is a common problem, especially among the elderly, adults with psychiatric or mental health problems, or those who live alone or with reluctant or incapable caregivers. In some cases, **passive neglect** may occur because an elderly or impaired spouse or partner is trying to take care of a patient and is unable to provide the care needed, but in other cases, **active neglect** reflects a lack of caring which may be considered negligence or abuse. Cases of neglect should be reported to the appropriate governmental agency, such as adult protective services. Indications of neglect include the following:

- Lack of assistive devices, such as a cane or walker, needed for mobility
- Misplaced or missing glasses or hearing aids
- Poor dental hygiene and dental care or missing dentures
- Patient left unattended for extended periods of time, sometimes confined to a bed or chair
- Patient left in soiled or urine- and feces-stained clothing
- Inadequate food, fluid, or nutrition, resulting in weight loss
- Inappropriate and unkempt clothing, such as no sweater or coat during the winter and dirty or torn clothing
- A dirty, messy environment

ELDERLY AND DISABLED NEGLECT AND ABUSE

The elderly and disabled are at risk for neglect and abuse when they have impaired mental processes or physical deficits that affect ADLs. They are also at risk when there are caregiver problems such as:

- High amount of stress
- Substance abuse
- Physical abusive or violent
- Emotionally unstable or with mental illness
- Dependency on the elderly or disabled person for money, emotional support, or physical support

The nurse should act to help a caregiver to cope more effectively to prevent abuse from occurring by providing an outlet for emotions and referring to resources. It's important to ask patients in private whether anyone prevents them from using medical assistive devices or refuses to help them with ADLs. However, many will not admit to abuse. If there are risk factors present or signs of abuse, the nurse must act to preserve the safety of the individual. Most states require the reporting of elder abuse and neglect. Assist the person in accessing resources in the community to improve their living situation.

DOMESTIC VIOLENCE

Men, women, elderly, children, and the disabled may all be victims of **domestic violence**. The violent person harms physically or sexually and uses threats and fear to maintain control of the victim. The violence does not improve unless the abuser gets intensive counseling. The abuser may promise not to do it again, but the violence usually gets more frequent and worsens over time. The nurse should ask all patients in private about abuse, neglect, and fear of a caretaker. If abuse is suspected or there are signs present, the state may require **reporting**:

- Give victims information about community hotlines, shelters, and resources.
- Urge them to set up a plan for escape for themselves and any children, complete with supplies in a location away from the home.
- Assure victims that they are not at fault and do not deserve the abuse.
- Try to empower them by helping them to realize that they do not have to take abuse and can find support to change the situation.
- Assessment of Domestic Violence

According to the guidelines of the Family Violence Prevention Fund, **assessment** for domestic violence should be done for all adolescent and adult patients, regardless of background or signs of abuse. While females are the most common victims, there are increasing reports of male victims of domestic violence, both in heterosexual and homosexual relationships. The person doing the assessment should be informed about domestic violence and be aware of risk factors and danger signs. The interview should be conducted in private (special accommodations may need to be made for children <3 years old). The nurse manager's office, bathrooms, and examining rooms should have information about domestic violence posted prominently. Brochures and information should be available to give to patients. Patients may present with a variety of physical complaints, such as headache, pain, palpitations, numbness, or pelvic pain. They are often depressed and may appear suicidal and may be isolated from friends and family. Victims of domestic violence often exhibit fear of spouse/partner, and may report injury inconsistent with symptoms.

STEPS TO IDENTIFYING VICTIMS OF DOMESTIC VIOLENCE

The **Family Violence Prevention Fund** has issued guidelines for identifying and assisting victims of domestic violence. There are 7 steps:

1. **Inquiry**: Non-judgmental questioning should begin with asking if the person has ever been abused—physically, sexually, or psychologically.
2. **Interview**: The person may exhibit signs of anxiety or fear and may blame himself or report that others believe he is abused. The person should be questioned if she is afraid for her life or for her children.
3. **Question**: If the person reports abuse, it's critical to ask if the person is in immediate danger or if the abuser is on the premises. The interviewer should ask if the person has been threatened. The history and pattern of abuse should be questioned, and if children are involved, whether the children are abused. Note: State laws vary, and in some states, it is mandatory to report if a child was present during an act of domestic violence as this is considered child abuse. The nurse must be aware of state laws regarding domestic and child abuse, and all nurses are mandatory reporters.
4. **Validate**: The interviewer should offer support and reassurance in a non-judgmental manner, telling the patient the abuse is not his or her fault.
5. **Give information**: While discussing facts about domestic violence and the tendency to escalate, the interviewer should provide brochures and information about safety planning. If the patient wants to file a complaint with the police, the interviewer should assist the person to place the call.
6. **Make referrals**: Information about state, local, and national organizations should be provided along with telephone numbers and contact numbers for domestic violence shelters.
7. **Document**: Record keeping should be legal, legible, and lengthy with a complete report and description of any traumatic injuries resulting from domestic violence. A body map may be used to indicate sites of injury, especially if there are multiple bruises or injuries.

INJURIES CONSISTENT WITH DOMESTIC VIOLENCE

There are a number of characteristic **injuries** that may indicate domestic violence, including ruptured eardrum; rectal/genital injury (burns, bites, or trauma); scrapes and bruises about the neck, face, head, trunk, arms; and cuts, bruises, and fractures of the face. The pattern of injuries associated with domestic violence is also often distinctive. The bathing-suit pattern involves injuries on parts of body that are usually covered with clothing as the perpetrator inflicts damage but hides evidence of abuse. Head and neck injuries (50%) are also common. Abusive injuries (rarely attributable to accidents) are common and include bites, bruises, rope and cigarette burns, and welts in the outline of weapons (belt marks). Bilateral injuries of arms/legs are often seen with domestic abuse. Defensive injuries are indicative of abuse.

Defensive injuries to the back of the body are often incurred as the victim crouches on the floor face down while being attacked. The soles of the feet may be injured from kicking at perpetrator. The ulnar aspect of hand or palm may be injured from blocking blows.

Theories of Human Growth and Development

ISSUES OF HUMAN DEVELOPMENT

Several issues of human development that are addressed by theory are described below:

- **Universality vs. context specificity**: Universality implies that all individuals will develop in the same way, no matter what culture they live in. Context Specificity implies that development will be influenced by the culture in which the individual lives.
- **Assumptions about human nature** (3 doctrines: original sin, innate purity, and tabula rasa):
  o Original sin says that children are inherently bad and must be taught to be good.
  o Innate purity says that children are inherently good.
  o Tabula rasa says that children are born without good or bad tendencies and can be taught right vs. wrong.
- **Behavioral consistency**: Children either behave in the same manner no matter what the situation or setting, or they change their behavior depending on the setting and who is interacting with them.
- **Nature vs. nurture**: Nature is the genetic influences on development. Nurture is the environment and social influences on development.
- **Continuity vs. discontinuity**: Continuity states that development progresses at a steady rate and the effects of change are cumulative. Discontinuity states that development progresses in a stair-step fashion and the effects of early development have no bearing on later development.
- **Passivity vs. activity**: Passivity refers to development being influenced by outside forces. Activity refers to development influenced by the child himself and how he responds to external forces.
- **Critical vs. sensitive period**: The critical period is that window of time when the child will be able to acquire new skills and behaviors. The sensitive period refers to a flexible time period when a child will be receptive to learning new skills, even if it is later than the norm.

DEVELOPMENTAL TASKS ACCORDING TO ERIKSON

The developmental tasks according to Erik Erikson:

- **Trust vs. Mistrust (Birth to 1 year)**: Trust, faith and optimism develop if the needs of warmth, food and love are met. If not, this can result in mistrust.
- **Autonomy vs. Shame/Doubt (Ages 1-3)**: The child desires independence in basic self-care tasks and wants choice. If independence is not encouraged, this can lead to doubt and shame. Independence develops self-control and willpower.
- **Initiative vs. Guilt (Ages 3-6)**: The child engages in self-directed play and starts activities without outside influence. Imaginative play and competition are introduced. This can lead to guilt or direction and purpose based on how this initiative is supportive.
- **Industry vs. Inferiority (Ages 6-12)**: The child values feeling capable and competent, and develops a sense of pride and self-worth. They desire to do what is right and good. Social interactions between peers becomes more important, and comparing achievements can result in feelings of pride or feelings of inferiority if not properly guided.
- **Identity vs. Role Confusion (Ages 12-18)**: Parents, teachers, peers, family members, church, culture, and ethnicity all role model and pressure youth to adopt certain behaviors. The task of adolescents is to discover their own identity.

13

- **Intimacy vs. Isolation (Ages 18-40)**: Young people learn to commit to another person in a love or family relationship. They learn the behavior required to maintain this relationship.
- **Generativity vs. Stagnation (Ages 40-65)**: Adults have many tasks when they try to find their own interests and niche in the work world. Family, community, and work roles are defined.
- **Integrity vs. Despair (Ages 65+)**: Older people ponder their life experiences to put them into perspective. They learn to accept the aging process and begin to think about their own death.

SIGMUND FREUD'S STAGES OF PSYCHOSEXUAL DEVELOPMENT

Sigmund Freud's stages of psychosexual development are listed and described below:

- **Oral stage (Birth to 1 year)**: obsessed with oral activities and must have these needs met for proper psychosocial development, very attached to mother.
- **Anal stage (Ages 1-3)**: masters toilet training.
- **Phallic stage (Ages 3-6)**: child focuses on childbirth and differences between the sexes, develops sexual obsession with parent of opposite sex (Oedipal complex-boy drawn to mother, Electra complex-girl drawn to father).
- **Latency stage (Ages 6-11)**: Oedipal or Electra complex wanes, focus is now socialization, begins to gravitate toward the same sex parent to learn appropriate gender roles.
- **Genital stage (Ages 12 and older)**: puberty, attracted to opposite sex, learns to relate to opposite gender and control sexual drive.

PIAGET'S THEORY OF COGNITIVE DEVELOPMENT

Piaget believed that development was progressive and followed a set pattern. He believed the child's environment, his interactions with others in that environment, and how the environment responds help to shape his cognitive development. There are **4 stages to Piaget's theory:**

- The **sensorimotor stage (birth to age 2)** is when the child learns to work toward a goal, the relationship between cause and effect, that objects still exist even though they cannot see them, and a sense of self.
- In the **preoperational stage (ages 2-7)** language skills develop, the child only sees his point of view, he does not think abstractly, and has a difficult time telling fact from fantasy.
- The **concrete operations stage (ages 7-11)** is when children begin to understand relationships between objects and events, learn to classify and use patterns, understand that some occurrences are reversible, and see other's points of view.
- The **formal operations stage (ages 12 years and older)** is the stage of abstract thinking, better reasoning skills, and forward thinking.

MASLOW'S HIERARCHY OF NEEDS

Maslow defined human motivation in terms of needs and wants. His **hierarchy of needs** is classically portrayed as a pyramid sitting on its base divided into horizontal layers. He theorized that, as humans fulfill the needs of one layer, their motivation turns to the layer above. The layers consist of (from bottom to top):

- **Physiological**: The need for air, fluid, food, shelter, warmth, and sleep.
- **Safety**: A safe place to live, a steady job, a society with rules and laws, protection from harm, and insurance or savings for the future.
- **Love/Belonging**: A network consisting of a significant other, family, friends, co-workers, religion, and community.
- **Esteem or self-respect**: The knowledge that you are a person who is successful and worthy of esteem, attention, status, and admiration.
- **Self-actualization**: The acceptance of your life, choices, and situation in life and the empathetic acceptance of others, as well as the feeling of independence and the joy of being able to express yourself freely and competently.

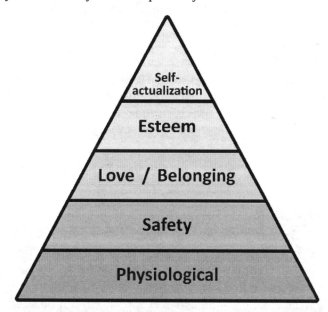

Review Video: **Maslow's Hierarchy of Needs**
Visit mometrix.com/academy and enter code: 461825

BEHAVIORAL THEORIES

Pavlov demonstrated classical conditioning when he found that a dog that would salivate when presented with food would also salivate when the person who normally fed him was present. He paired a bell ringing with the feeding and found that after a time, the dog would also salivate to the ringing of the bell. Consequently, his theory was that learning takes place when a behavior can be produced in response to something totally unrelated to that behavior.

Skinner demonstrated operant conditioning when he found that behavior can be changed depending on the response given to the behavior. If the response to the behavior was positive (praise, a hug) then the behavior would continue or increase in frequency. If the response was negative (a frown, words of criticism) then the behavior would decrease in frequency or cease altogether.

BIOPSYCHOSOCIAL THEORY OF PATIENT CARE

The biopsychosocial theory of patient care recognizes that **biology, psychology, and social circumstances** all interact in the development of an illness, the patient's perception of the illness, and the patient's ability to make a good recovery. In the biopsychosocial care model, a multidisciplinary healthcare team, including nurses, mental health professionals, social workers, and physicians, work together to address all aspects of a patient's health issue—the medical problem, psychological state, and social, cultural, and economic situation—in order to find an integrated solution. For example, adding stress-reduction, exercise, and nutritional programs to the standard medical treatment protocol for cardiovascular disease patients has been shown to be more effective. Many patients with chronic diseases or conditions may benefit from support groups that provide social and psychological benefits that may enhance the effects of drug therapy and surgery.

BIOLOGICAL THEORIES OF AGING

There are a number of biological theories of aging:

- **Wearing down**: The body is compared to a machine that simply begins to wear down over time because of the damage caused by years of use.
- **Autoimmune reaction**: The body develops an autoimmune reaction against itself with aging, causing damage and destruction to tissues.
- **Free radical accumulation**: Chemicals that bring about aging accumulate in the body.
- **Cellular programming**: The cells of every organism have a pre-determined programmed life expectancy beyond which one cannot survive.
- **Mutation**: Mutations within the organism occur over time and these eventually make changes that are incompatible with life.
- **Homeostasis**: Over time, the body is unable to maintain stable levels of necessary chemicals in the body.

SELYE'S THEORY OF ADAPTATION

Selye developed a theory of adaptation concerning a person's physiologic response to stress called the general adaptation syndrome. This syndrome starts with the classic "fight or flight" response of the body to physiologic stress. Catecholamines are released and the adrenal cortical response begins. This is called the **alarm response** and is short-lived. This immediate response allows the person to respond quickly to stress. Since the alarm response cannot be sustained without resulting in death, the body next shifts into the **resistance stage**. Some cortisol is still being released as the body begins to adapt to the stressor. If the stressor persists, the body becomes exhausted. Changes then occur to the cardiovascular, gastrointestinal, and immune systems and death can occur. The **exhaustion stage** does not always occur in response to most life stressors. As the body ages, it loses some of its resistance and ability to adapt to stress. This results in exhaustion and death in the elderly more easily than it does in younger people.

Communication

Therapeutic Relationships

THERAPEUTIC COMMUNICATION

FACILITATING COMMUNICATION

Therapeutic communication begins with respect for the patient/family and the assumption that all communication, verbal and nonverbal, has meaning. Listening must be done empathetically. The following are some techniques that facilitate communication.

Introduction:

- Make a personal introduction and use the patient's name: "Mrs. Brown, I am Susan Williams, your nurse."

Encouragement:

- Use an open-ended opening statement: "Is there anything you'd like to discuss?"
- Acknowledge comments: "Yes," and "I understand."
- Allow silence and observe nonverbal behavior rather than trying to force conversation. Ask for clarification if statements are unclear.
- Reflect statements back (use sparingly): Patient: "I hate this hospital." Nurse: "You hate this hospital?"

Empathy:

- Make observations: "You are shaking," and "You seem worried."
- Recognize feelings:
  - Patient: "I want to go home."
  - Nurse: "It must be hard to be away from your home and family."
- Provide information as honestly and completely as possible about condition, treatment, and procedures and respond to the patient's questions and concerns.

Exploration:

- Verbally express implied messages:
  - Patient: "This treatment is too much trouble."
  - Nurse: "You think the treatment isn't helping you?"
- Explore a topic but allow the patient to terminate the discussion without further probing: "I'd like to hear how you feel about that."

17

Orientation:

- Indicate reality:
  - Patient: "Someone is screaming."
  - Nurse: "That sound was an ambulance siren."
- Comment on distortions without directly agreeing or disagreeing:
  - Patient: "That nurse promised I didn't have to walk again."
  - Nurse: "Really? That's surprising because the doctor ordered physical therapy twice a day."

Collaboration:

- Work together to achieve better results: "Maybe if we talk about this, we can figure out a way to make the treatment easier for you."

Validation:

- Seek validation: "Do you feel better now?" or "Did the medication help you breathe better?"

AVOIDING NON-THERAPEUTIC COMMUNICATION

While using therapeutic communication is important, it is equally important to avoid interjecting **non-therapeutic communication**, which can block effective communication. *Avoid the following:*

- Meaningless clichés: "Don't worry. Everything will be fine." "Isn't it a nice day?"
- Providing advice: "You should…" or "The best thing to do is…." It's better when patients ask for advice to provide facts and encourage the patient to reach a decision.
- Inappropriate approval that prevents the patient from expressing true feeling or concerns:
  - Patient: "I shouldn't cry about this."
  - Nurse: "That's right! You're an adult!"
- Asking for an explanation of behavior that is not directly related to patient care and requires analysis and explanation of feelings: "Why are you so upset?"
- Agreeing with rather than accepting and responding to patient's statements can make it difficult for the patient to change his or her statement or opinion later: "I agree with you," or "You are right."
- Making negative judgments: "You should stop arguing with the nurses."
- Devaluing the patient's feelings: "Everyone gets upset at times."
- Disagreeing directly: "That can't be true," or "I think you are wrong."
- Defending against criticism: "The doctor is not being rude; he's just very busy today."
- Changing the subject to avoid dealing with uncomfortable topics;
  - Patient: "I'm never going to get well."
  - Nurse: "Your family will be here in just a few minutes."
- Making inappropriate literal responses, even as a joke, especially if the patient is at all confused or having difficulty expressing ideas:
  - Patient: "There are bugs crawling under my skin."
  - Nurse: "I'll get some bug spray,"
- Challenging the patient to establish reality often just increases confusion and frustration:
  - "If you were dying, you wouldn't be able to yell and kick!"

COMMUNICATING WITH PATIENTS WITH DISABILITIES

Guidelines for communicating with individuals with disabilities:

- Do not assume that the person with disabilities also has impaired cognition.
- Always treat the person with respect and dignity.
- Use first names with the patient if asked to do so, but start out formally as with any patient.
- Offer to shake hands even when a prosthesis is present.
- Be patient if communication is impaired.
- Offer assistance, but allow the patient to tell you what is helpful; otherwise don't assist.
- When a wheelchair is used, sit down so the patient does not have to strain their neck to speak with you.
- If providing directions, consider the obstacles that may be in the way and assist the person to find an appropriate way around them.

COMMUNICATION WITH PATIENTS WITH COGNITIVE DISABILITIES

The person with cognitive disabilities may be easily distracted, so verbal communication should be attempted in a quiet area:

- Address people with dignity and respect.
- Do not try to discuss abstract ideas but stick with concrete topics.
- Keep words and sentences very simple and try rephrasing when necessary. People may have difficulty in distinguishing your spoken words and deriving the meaning from them.
- Be very patient with people's attempts to speak to you since they may have difficulty in processing thoughts and changing them into spoken words.
- Use objects around you and gestures to illustrate your words since the patient may also use pointing and gesturing when unable to find the words to communicate with you. The person may prefer written communication, although some may be unable to read.
- Use touch to convey your regard during communication, as this is recognized by the patient as reassurance of your care and concern for them.
- Give a few instructions at a time as to not overwhelm them.

COMMUNICATING WITH DEAF OR HEARING-IMPAIRED PATIENTS

Communicating with a person with deafness or hearing impairment:

- Try to communicate in a quiet environment if possible.
- Wave or touch the person to let him or her know you are trying to communicate.
- Determine the method the person uses to communicate: sign language, lip reading, hearing devices, or writing.
- Fingerspell or use some signs if able to do so.
- Address the person directly when you speak even though the person may be looking at an interpreter or your lips.
- Look at the person as the interpreter tells you what was said.
- Speak slowly so the interpreter can keep up with you.
- If the person reads lips, face the person and speak clearly and normally, using normal volume.
- If writing a communication, do not speak while writing.
- Do not be afraid to check that the person understands you, and ask questions if you do not understand the person.

COMMUNICATION WITH PEOPLE WITH LOW VISION OR BLINDNESS

Communicating with a person with low vision or blindness:

- Greet the person with low vision or blindness, identifying yourself and others present.
- Always say goodbye when you are leaving.
- Alert the person to written communications, such as warning signs or printed notices.
- Face the person and touch briefly on the arm to let the person know you are speaking to him or her if you are in a group.
- Speak at normal loudness.
- Make any directions given specific in terms of the length of walk and obstacles, such as stairs.
- Use the position of hands on a clock face to give directions (potatoes at 3 o'clock) as well as using *right* or *left*.
- Mention sounds that the person may hear in transit or on arrival at a destination.
- Do not be afraid to use the word *see*, as the person will probably use it as well.

COMMUNICATING WITH A PATIENT ON A VENTILATOR

When a patient on a ventilator is conscious, he or she may still be able to communicate by blinking, nodding, shaking the head, or pointing to a picture or word board:

- If the person is able to write, try to reposition the IV line to leave the dominant hand free to communicate.
- Discuss the need for communication with the physician and ask if a valve or an electric larynx can be used to permit speech.
- Help the patient practice lip reading of single words.
- Remember the patient's glasses or hearing aids when attempting to communicate.
- Enlist the aid of a speech therapist if there is frustration on the part of the patient and family due to communication difficulty.

COMMUNICATING WITH PERSONS WITH SPEECH PROBLEMS DUE TO A STROKE

Methods to communicate with stroke patients with speech problems:

- **Dysarthria**: Patients have problems forming the words to speak them aloud. Give them time to communicate, offer them a picture board or other means of communicating, and give encouragement to family members who are frustrated with the difficulty of trying to communicate.
- **Expressive aphasia**: The patients' efforts at speech come out garbled when they try to say sentences, but single words may be clear. Encourage the patients to try to write and to practice the sounds of the alphabet. Resist the urge to finish sentences for the patients.
- **Receptive aphasia**: The patients have a problem comprehending the speech they hear. Communicate in simple terms and speak slowly. Test comprehension of the written word as an alternative method of communication.
- **Global aphasia**: The patient has both receptive and expressive aphasia. Use simple, clear, slow speech augmented by pictures and gestures.

COMMUNICATION PROBLEMS OF PATIENTS WITH PARKINSON'S DISEASE

Parkinson's disease causes problems with speaking in the majority (75-90%) of patients. The reason for this is not clear but may relate to increasing rigidity and changes in movement. Speech is often very low-pitched or hoarse, given in a monotone and with a soft voice. Speech production may decrease because of the effort required to speak. **Speech therapy** can develop exercises for the patient that can assist them in remembering to speak slowly and carefully, as patients are not always aware that their **communication** is impaired:

- Allow time for the patient to communicate, asking for repetition if you do not understand the message.
- Help family by teaching ways to facilitate communication with the patient and encouraging them to assist the patient to do the exercises provided by the therapist.
- If speech volume is very low, suggest amplification devices that can be obtained through speech therapy.

COMMUNICATION WITH PATIENTS WITH PSYCHIATRIC PROBLEMS

Persons with psychiatric disorders appreciate being addressed with respect, dignity, and honesty:

- Speak simply and clearly, repeating as necessary.
- Encourage patients to discuss their concerns regarding treatment and medications to improve compliance.
- Use good eye contact and be attentive to your body language messages.
- Be alert, but unless the person is known to be violent, try to relax and listen to them.
- Don't try to avoid words or phrases pertaining to psychiatric problems, but if you do say something inappropriate, apologize honestly to the patient.
- Offer patients outlets for their thoughts and feelings.
- Learn more about their disorder and ways to use therapeutic communication to help them with their problem, such as re-orienting them as needed.

CULTURAL COMPETENCE

Different cultures view health and illness from very different perspectives, and patients often come from a mix of many cultures, so the nurse must be not only accepting of cultural differences but must be sensitive and aware. There are a number of characteristics that are important for a nurse to have **cultural competence**:

- **Appreciating diversity**: This must be grounded in information about other cultures and understanding of their value systems.
- **Assessing own cultural perspectives**: Self-awareness is essential to understanding potential biases.
- **Understanding intercultural dynamics**: This must include understanding ways in which cultures cooperate, differ, communicate, and reach understanding.
- **Recognizing institutional culture**: Each institutional unit (hospital, clinic, office) has an inherent set of values that may be unwritten but is accepted by the staff.
- **Adapting patient service to diversity**: This is the culmination of cultural competence as it is the point of contact between cultures.

RELIGIOUS OBJECTIONS TO TREATMENT

JEHOVAH'S WITNESSES

Jehovah's Witnesses have traditionally shunned transfusions and blood products as part of their religious beliefs. In 2004, the *Watchtower,* a Jehovah's Witness publication, presented a guide for members. When medical care indicates the need for blood transfusion or blood products and the patient and/or family members are practicing Jehovah's Witnesses, this may present a conflict. It's important to approach the patient/family with full information and reasons for the transfusion or blood components without being judgmental, allowing them to express their feelings. In fact, studies show that while adults often refuse transfusions for themselves, they frequently allow their children to receive blood products, so one should never assume that an individual would refuse blood products based on the religion alone. Jehovah's Witnesses can receive fractionated blood cells, thus allowing hemoglobin-based blood substitutes. The following guidelines are provided to church members:

Basic **blood standards for Jehovah's Witnesses**:

- **Not acceptable**: Whole blood: red cells, white cells, platelets, plasma.
- **Acceptable**: Fractions from red cells, white cells, platelets, and plasma.

CHRISTIAN SCIENTISTS

Christian Science, a religion developed by Mary Baker Eddy in 1879, promotes the belief that sickness is most effectively treated through prayer alone. While Christian Scientists do not avoid all medical interventions, their beliefs are conservative regarding medical treatment. Most notably, Christian Scientists, for the most part, do not believe in vaccinations and may only agree to such if required by law, as they do acknowledge the importance of community health. They have widely appreciated the use of exemptions from mandatory vaccines, but as these exemptions have become more limited, religious leaders have given their members the right to decide upon vaccinations.

CULTURAL CHARACTERISTICS

HISPANIC PATIENTS

Many areas of the country have large populations of Hispanics and Hispanic Americans. As always, it's important to recognize that cultural generalizations don't always apply to individuals. Recent immigrants, especially, have cultural needs that the nurse must understand:

- Many Hispanics are Catholic and may like the nurse to make arrangements for a priest to visit.
- Large extended families may come to visit to support the patient and family, so patients should receive clear explanations about how many visitors are allowed, but some flexibility may be required.
- Language barriers may exist as some may have limited or no English skills, so translation services should be available around the clock.
- Hispanic culture encourages outward expressions of emotions, so family may react strongly to news about a patient's condition, and people who are ill may expect some degree of pampering, so extra attention to the patient/family members may alleviate some of their anxiety.

Caring for Hispanic and Hispanic American patients requires understanding of cultural differences:

- Some immigrant Hispanics have very little formal education, so medical information may seem very complex and confusing, and they may not understand the implications or need for follow-up care.
- Hispanic culture perceives time with more flexibility than American culture, so if parents need to be present at a particular time, the nurse should specify the exact time (1:30 PM) and explain the reason rather than saying something more vague, such as "after lunch."
- People may appear to be unassertive or unable to make decisions when they are simply showing respect to the nurse by being deferent.
- In traditional families, the males make decisions, so a woman waits for the father or other males in the family to make decisions about treatment or care.
- Families may choose to use folk medicines instead of Western medical care or may combine the two.
- Children and young women are often sheltered and are taught to be respectful to adults, so they may not express their needs openly.

MIDDLE EASTERN PATIENTS

There are considerable cultural differences among Middle Easterners, but religious beliefs about the segregation of males and females are common. It's important to remember that segregating the female is meant to protect her virtue. Female nurses have low status in many countries because they violate this segregation by touching male bodies, so parents may not trust or show respect for the nurse who is caring for their family member. Additionally, male patients may not want to be cared for by female nurses or doctors, and families may be very upset at a female being cared for by a male nurse or physician. When possible, these cultural traditions should be accommodated:

- In Middle Eastern countries, males make decisions, so issues for discussion or decision should be directed to males, such as the father or spouse, and males may be direct in stating what they want, sometimes appearing demanding.
- If a male nurse must care for a female patient, then the family should be advised that *personal care* (such as bathing) will be done by a female while the medical treatments will be done by the male nurse.

Caring for Middle Eastern patients requires understanding of cultural differences:

- Families may practice strict dietary restrictions, such as avoiding pork and requiring that animals be killed in a ritual manner, so vegetarian or kosher meals may be required.
- People may have language difficulties requiring a translator, and same-sex translators should be used if at all possible.
- Families may be accompanied by large extended families that want to be kept informed and whom patients consult before decisions are made.
- Most medical care is provided by female relatives, so educating the family about patient care should be directed at females (with female translators if necessary).
- Outward expressions of grief are considered as showing respect for the dead.
- Middle Eastern families often offer gifts to caregivers. Small gifts (candy) that can be shared should be accepted graciously, but for other gifts, the families should be advised graciously that accepting gifts is against hospital policy.
- Middle Easterners often require less personal space and may stand very close.

ASIAN PATIENTS

There are considerable differences among different Asian populations, so cultural generalizations may not apply to all, but nurses caring for Asian patients should be aware of common cultural attitudes and behaviors:

- Nurses and doctors are viewed with respect, so traditional Asian families may expect the nurse to remain authoritative and to give directions and may not question, so the nurse should ensure that they understand by having them review material or give demonstrations and should provide explanations clearly, anticipating questions that the family might have but may not articulate.
- Disagreeing is considered impolite. "Yes" may only mean that the person is heard, not that they agree with the person. When asked if they understand, they may indicate that they do even when they clearly do not so as not to offend the nurse.
- Asians may avoid eye contact as an indication of respect. This is especially true of children in relation to adults and of younger adults in relation to elders.

Caring for Asian patients requires understanding of cultural differences:

- Patients/families may not show outward expressions of feelings/grief, sometimes appearing passive. They also avoid public displays of affection. This does not mean that they don't feel, just that they don't show their feelings.
- Families often hide illness and disabilities from others and may feel ashamed about illness.
- Terminal illness is often hidden from the patient, so families may not want patients to know they are dying or seriously ill.
- Families may use cupping, pinching, or applying pressure to injured areas, and this can leave bruises that may appear as abuse, so when bruises are found, the family should be questioned about alternative therapy before assumptions are made.
- Patients may be treated with traditional herbs.
- Families may need translators because of poor or no English skills.
- In traditional Asian families, males are authoritative and make the decisions.

IMPACT OF CULTURE AND RELIGION ON DIETARY PREFERENCES

When performing a dietary assessment, the nurse should remember that culture and religion might dictate which foods and spices are used. The manner in which food is prepared, cooked, and served may also be specified. The utensils used at the meal as well as the persons who may eat together may be important. Mealtimes and required fasts should be determined. Holidays may be accompanied by particular foods. Alcohol (including extracts made with alcohol) and caffeine may be prohibited. The culture may also consider obesity a sign of affluence and success. The nurse should evaluate the foods that are eaten in light of the patient's medical condition. The patient may not wish to eat the usual hospital fare and may need to have a special diet prepared or food brought from home. The nurse can guide the patient and family to foods that are acceptable and within the patient's requirements for health.

Education Theory

BANDURA'S THEORY OF SOCIAL LEARNING

In the 1970s, Bandura proposed the **theory of social learning,** in which he posited that learning develops from observing, organizing, and rehearsing behavior that has been modeled. Bandura believed that people are more likely to adopt the behavior if they value the outcomes, if the outcomes have functional value, and if the person modeling the behavior is similar to the learner and is admired because of status. Behavior is the result of observation of behavioral, environmental, and cognitive interactions. There are **4 conditions required for modeling**:

- **Attention**: The degree of attention paid to modeling can depend on many variables (physical, social, and environmental).
- **Retention**: People's ability to retain models depends on symbolic coding, creating mental images, organizing thoughts, and rehearsing (mentally or physically).
- **Reproduction**: The ability to reproduce a model depends on physical and mental capabilities.
- **Motivation**: Motivation may derive from past performances, rewards, or vicarious modeling.

TRANSTHEORETICAL MODEL OF CHANGE

The Transtheoretical Model of Change puts forth concepts applicable to the process of educating patients and their family members. The **stages of the Transtheoretical Model of Change** include the following:

1. The first stage is **precontemplation**. At this point, the patient is not aware of any need for a change in the health behavior.
2. In the next stage, **contemplation**, the patient begins to realize why the change may be necessary after recognizing that the health behavior in question is unhealthy and weighing the consequences of continuing this behavior.
3. During the stage of **preparation**, the patient imagines making the change at a future time, and starts to formulate a plan to do so.
4. The **action** stage occurs when the patient makes specific modifications in health behavior and begins to note the resulting positive changes.
5. During the **maintenance** stage, the patient is able to implement the change over time by utilizing strategies to prevent a return to previously unhealthy behaviors.
6. **Termination** is the stage at which a patient has incorporated the changed behavior into daily functioning, and the patient will not resume the previous unhealthy behavior.

KURT LEWIN

FORCE FIELD ANALYSIS

Force field analysis was designed by Kurt Lewin, a social psychologist, to analyze both the driving forces and the restraining forces for change:

- **Driving forces** instigate and promote change, such as leaders, incentives, and competition.
- **Restraining forces** resist change, such as poor attitudes, hostility, inadequate equipment, or insufficient funds.

The educator can use this force field analysis diagram to discuss variables related to a proposed change in process:

- Write the proposed change in the center column.
- Brainstorm and list driving forces and opposed restraining forces. Score the forces. (When driving and restraining forces are in balance, this is a state of equilibrium or the status quo.)
- Discuss the value of the proposed change.
- Develop a plan to diminish or eliminate restraining forces.

LEWIN'S MODEL OF CHANGE THEORY

Lewin's model of change theory may be used to help some patients make decisions for change. The nurse can educate the patient about the need for change and assist with making alterations in behavior or thoughts in order to better facilitate change; however, only the patient can truly implement the change permanently. Lewin's concept of change theory involves a three-part process:

- **Unfreezing** is the part of the model in which the patient becomes open to change, sees a need for it, and removes the boundaries inhibiting change.
- The patient then makes the **actual change** according to expected outcomes and goals.
- Finally, **refreezing** is the process of maintaining the change so that it becomes a habit, and one that the patient is likely to uphold for a long period of time.

Lewin's theory also involves either driving forces or restraining forces. Driving forces are those outside measures that support the change, while restraining forces inhibit success in implementing the change.

Principles of Education

PRINCIPLES OF ADULT LEARNING

Adults have a wealth of life and/or employment experiences. Their attitudes toward education may vary considerably. There are, however, some **principles of adult learning** and typical characteristics of adult learners that an instructor should consider when planning strategies for teaching parents, families, or staff.

- Practical and goal-oriented:
  - Provide overviews or summaries and examples.
  - Use collaborative discussions with problem-solving exercises.
  - Remain organized with the goal in mind.
- Self-directed:
  - Provide active involvement, asking for input.
  - Allow different options toward achieving the goal.
  - Give them responsibilities.
- Knowledgeable:
  - Show respect for their life experiences/ education.
  - Validate their knowledge and ask for feedback.
  - Relate new material to information with which they are familiar.
- Relevancy-oriented:
  - Explain how information will be applied.
  - Clearly identify objectives.
- Motivated:
  - Provide certificates of professional advancement and/or continuing education credit for staff when possible.

> **Review Video: Adult Learning Processes and Theories**
> Visit mometrix.com/academy and enter code: 638453

LEARNING STYLES

Not all people are aware of their preferred **learning style.** A range of teaching materials and methods that relate to all three major learning preferences (visual, auditory, and kinesthetic) and that are appropriate for different ages should be available. Part of assessment for teaching involves choosing the right approach based on observation and feedback. Often presenting learners with different options gives a clue to their preferred learning style. Some people have a combined learning style.

Visual learners learn best by seeing and reading:

- Provide written directions, picture guides, or demonstrate procedures. Use charts and diagrams.
- Provide photos, videos.

Auditory learners learn best by listening and talking:

- Explain procedures while demonstrating and have the learner repeat.
- Plan extra time to discuss and answer questions.
- Provide audiotapes.

Kinesthetic learners learn best by handling, doing, and practicing:

- Provide hands-on experience throughout teaching.
- Encourage handling of supplies and equipment.
- Allow the learner to demonstrate.
- Minimize instructions and allow the person to explore equipment and procedures.

BLOOM'S TAXONOMY

Bloom's taxonomy outlines behaviors that are necessary for learning and that can be applied to healthcare. The theory describes 3 types of learning.

Cognitive: Learning and gaining intellectual skills to master 6 categories of effective learning.

- Knowledge
- Comprehension
- Application
- Analysis
- Synthesis
- Evaluation

Affective: Recognizing 5 categories of feelings and values from simple to complex. This is slower to achieve than cognitive learning.

- **Receiving phenomena**: Accepting need to learn
- **Responding to phenomena**: Taking active part in care
- **Valuing**: Understanding value of becoming independent in care
- **Organizing values**: Understanding how surgery/treatment has improved life
- **Internalizing values**: Accepting condition as part of life, being consistent and self-reliant

Psychomotor: Mastering 7 categories of motor skills necessary for independence. This follows a progression from simple to complex.

- **Perception**: Uses sensory information to learn tasks
- **Set**: Shows willingness to perform tasks
- **Guided response**: Follows directions
- **Mechanism**: Does specific tasks
- **Complex overt response**: Displays competence in self-care
- **Adaptation**: Modifies procedures as needed
- **Origination**: Creatively deals with problems

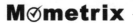

APPROACHES TO TEACHING

There are many approaches to teaching, and the educator must prepare, present, and coordinate a wide range of educational workshops, lectures, discussions, and one-on-one instructions on any chosen topic. All types of classes will be needed, depending upon the purpose and material:

- **Educational workshops** are usually conducted with small groups, allowing for maximal participation. They are especially good for demonstrations and practice sessions.
- **Lectures** are often used for more academic or detailed information that may include questions and answers but limits discussion. An effective lecture should include some audiovisual support.
- **Discussions** are best with small groups so that people can actively participate. This is a good method for problem solving.
- **One-on-one instruction** is especially helpful for targeted instruction in procedures for individuals.
- **Online learning modules** are good for independent learners.

Participants should be asked to evaluate the presentations in the forms of surveys or suggestions, but ultimately the program is evaluated in terms of patient outcomes.

TEACHING TECHNIQUES

There are many teaching techniques the nurse can utilize when educating patients. The nurse can demonstrate skills repeatedly when teaching and then allow the patient as much time as needed to practice the skill. The nurse should use equipment that will be available in the home and provide written instructions that can be referred to later if needed. Encouraging discussion of the information helps the patient understand and clarify. Discussion also allows the patient to vent emotions about the disease and the learning process, and to assimilate the information so that a change in behavior can result. Discussion provides feedback to the patient and encouragement to continue learning. Teaching groups of people may be appropriate when there are others who require the same information. The members can support each other with encouragement, empathy, and camaraderie, although some patients will not learn well in groups and will need individual teaching. Groups must be followed up with on an individual basis to give the chance to clarify information, to evaluate the level of learning and goal achievement, and to alter the learning plan as needed for each person.

INSTRUCTION GROUP SIZES

Both one-on-one instruction and group instruction have a place in patient/family education.

- **One-on-one instruction** is the most costly for an institution because it is time intensive. However, it allows the patient and family more interaction with the nurse instructor and allows them to have more control over the process by asking questions or having the instructor repeat explanations or demonstrations. One-on-one instruction is especially valuable when patients and families must learn particular skills, such as managing dialysis, or if confidentiality is important.
- **Group instruction** is the less costly because the needs of a number of people can be met at one time. Group presentations are more planned and usually scheduled for a particular time period (an hour, for example), so patients and families have less control. Questioning is usually more limited and may be done only at the end. Group instruction allows patients/families with similar health problems to interact. Group instruction is especially useful for general types of instruction, such as managing diet or other lifestyle issues.

RESOURCES TO USE WHEN TEACHING PATIENTS AND THEIR FAMILIES

Many hospitals that find the need to repeatedly teach the same information to patients and families prepare brochures or other written materials or teaching videos that are available for use. The nurse should review material first and make notes specific to the patient. The nurse should also watch the video with the patient and discuss it afterwards. Written materials can augment lecture and demonstrations and are useful for the patient to keep for later reference.

There are also commercial materials that can be used, provided by various drug or equipment companies. **Teaching resources** are available online from the National Institutes of Health and other reputable sources. The nurse can use these prepared materials whenever possible to save time for actual teaching but must remember to customize them to the patient. They help provide pictures, colors, and interesting features that keep the patient's interest in learning alive. There are also many books, groups, and websites that the patient should be made aware of for resources after discharge.

READABILITY

Studies have indicated that learning is more effective if oral presentations and/or demonstrations are supplemented with reading materials, such as handouts. **Readability** (the grade level of the material) is a concern because many patients and families may have limited English skills or low literacy, and it can be difficult for the nurse to assess people's reading level. The average American reads effectively at the 6th to 8th grade level (regardless of education achieved), but many health education materials have a much higher readability level. Additionally, research indicates that even people with much higher reading skills learn medical and health information most effectively when the material is presented at the 6th to 8th grade readability level. Therefore, patient education materials (and consent forms) should not be written at higher than 6th to 8th grade level. Readability index calculators are available on the internet to give an approximation of grade level and difficulty for those preparing materials without expertise in teaching reading.

VIDEOS

Videos are a useful adjunct to teaching as they reduce the time needed for one-on-one instruction (increasing cost-effectiveness). Passive presentation of **videos**, such as in the waiting area, has little value, but focused viewing in which the nurse discusses the purpose of the video presentation prior to viewing and then is available for discussion after viewing can be very effective. Patients and/or families are often nervous about learning patient care and are unsure of their abilities, so they may not focus completely when the nurse is presenting information. Allowing the patients/families to watch a video demonstration or explanation first and allowing them to stop or review the video presentation can help them to grasp the fundamentals before they have to apply them, relieving some of the anxiety they may be experiencing. Videos are much more effective than written materials for those with low literacy or poor English skills. The nurse should always be available to answer questions and discuss the material after the patients/families finish viewing.

LEARNING CONTRACT

In order to be compliant with a therapeutic regimen, the patient needs information about the disease, the purpose of medications and treatments, and side effects and complications to watch for. A written **learning contract** organizes this information into specific learning goals, demonstrates the importance of the information, and ensures that all pertinent information is taught. Others on the healthcare team can note patient progress and easily determine what to teach next. The patient has a written plan to follow as well.

The learning contract should take into consideration the patient's age, sex, cultural and religious values, and educational level achieved. One must consider the patient's financial status, socio-economic status, living situation, and support network. The complex nature of a therapeutic regimen combined with distracters such as side effects, pain, denial, and fear can weaken the patient's resolve to maintain compliance. One must evaluate the patient's attitudes towards healthcare, coping mechanisms, and motivation and provide reinforcement as needed.

READINESS TO LEARN

The patient/family's readiness to learn should be assessed because if they are not ready, instruction is of little value. Often readiness is indicated when the patient/family asks questions or shows and interest in procedures. There are a number of factors related to readiness to learn:

- **Physical factors:** There are a number of physical factors than can affect ability. Manual dexterity may be required to complete a task, and this varies by age and condition. Hearing or vision deficits may impact a person's ability to learn. Complex tasks may be too difficult for some because of weakness or cognitive impairment, and modifications of the environment may be needed. Health status, age, and gender may all impact the ability to learn.
- **Experience:** People's experience with learning can vary widely and is affected by their ability to cope with changes, their personal goals, motivation to learn, and cultural background. People may have widely divergent ideas about what constitutes illness and/or treatment. Lack of English skills may make learning difficult and prevent people from asking questions.
- **Mental/emotional status:** The external support system and internal motivation may impact readiness. Anxiety, fear, or depression about one's condition can make learning very difficult because the patient/family cannot focus on learning, so the nurse must spend time to reassure the patient/family and wait until they are emotionally more receptive.
- **Knowledge/education:** The knowledge base of the patient/family, their cognitive ability, and their learning styles all affect their readiness to learn. The nurse should always begin by assessing what knowledge the patient/family already has about their disease, condition, or treatment and then build form that base. People with little medical experience may lack knowledge of basic medical terminology, interfering with their ability and readiness to learn.

EDUCATIONAL GOALS, OBJECTIVES, AND PLANS

Once a topic for performance improvement education has been chosen, then goals, measurable objectives with strategies, and lesson plans must be developed. A class should stay focused on one topic rather than trying to cover many. For example:

Goal: Increase compliance with hand hygiene standards in ICU.

Objectives:

- Develop series of posters and fliers by June 1.
- Observe 100% compliance with hand hygiene standards at 2 weeks, 1-month, and 2-month intervals after training is completed.

Strategies: Conduct 4 classes at different times over a one-week period, May 25-31.

- Place posters in all nursing units, staff rooms, and utility rooms by January 3.
- Develop slide show presentation for class and provide online access to the presentation for all staff by May 25.
- Utilize handwashing kits.

Lesson plans: Discussion period: Why do we need 100% compliance?

- Slide show: The case for hand hygiene
- Discussion: What did you learn?
- Demonstration and activities to show effectiveness
- Handwashing technique

LEARNER OUTCOMES

When the quality professional plans an educational offering, whether it be a class, an online module, a workshop, or educational materials, the professional should identify **learner outcomes,** which should be conveyed to the learners from the very beginning so that they are aware of the expectations. The subject matter of the educational material and the learner outcomes should be directly related. For example, if the quality professional is giving a class on decontamination of the environment, then a learner outcome might be: "Identify the difference between disinfectants and antiseptics." There may be one or multiple learner outcomes, but part of the assessment at the end of the learning experience should be to determine if, in fact, the learner outcomes have been achieved. A survey of whether or not the learners felt that they had achieved the learner outcomes can give valuable feedback and guidance to the quality professional.

IMPLEMENTATION AND EVALUATION OF TEACHING PLAN

Implementation and evaluation of the teaching plan includes:

- Follow teaching plan but be flexible and alter plan to suit the patient's learning needs.
- Work with a healthcare team to follow the teaching plan and ensure consistency in teaching methods as well as coordinate efforts and take responsibility for altering the plan and evaluating learning to meet goals.
- Monitor patient's motivational level, encourage with positive feedback as needed, and record patient responses to teaching and changes in behaviors as a result of all teaching sessions.
- Use tools, such as checklists, rating scales, observed behavior, written tests, and the nature of the questions from the patient when evaluating the effectiveness of the teaching plan in reaching the patient's goals for learning.
- Evaluate the plan after each session and at the end.

Communicate information taught and patient learning to any home health or community nurses involved. They can then continue the patient's teaching by evaluating behavior in the home and continuing to address learning needs as they arise.

EVALUATING EFFECTIVENESS OF EDUCATION

Education, like all interventions, must be evaluated for **effectiveness**. Two determinants of effectiveness include:

- **Behavior modification** involves thorough observation and measurement, identifying behavior that needs to be changed and then planning and instituting interventions to modify that behavior. The nurse can use a variety of techniques, including demonstrations of appropriate behavior, reinforcement, and monitoring until new behavior is adopted consistently. This is especially important when longstanding procedures and habits of behavior are changed.
- **Compliance rates** are often determined by observation, which should be done at intervals and on multiple occasions, but with patients, this may depend on self-reports. Outcomes is another measure of compliance; that is, if education is intended to improve patient health and reduce risk factors and that occurs, it is a good indication that there is compliance. Compliance rates are calculated by determining the number of events/procedures and degree of compliance.

TEACHING ELDERLY PATIENTS

The elderly patient's level of functioning must be assessed before teaching. Cognitive abilities and mental functioning may be affected by illness and aging:

- Short-term memory loss can affect the amount of material retained.
- Concentration may be decreased.
- Reaction time is delayed.
- Color discrimination, general vision, and hearing may be decreased.

The nurse should **pace** the teaching accordingly and **tailor** materials for any deficits. Family should be present for teaching if possible, to help the patient to remember key points after discharge. Large print on non-glare paper that is easy to read should be used. The nurse should use color-coding cues only if colors are easily perceived. The learning environment must be quiet and comfortable with no distractions or interruptions.

- Repeat information numerous times and allow the patient as much practice time as needed.
- Use audio-visual aids to reinforce information given verbally.
- Face the patient when speaking and encourage him/her to use hearing devices if used.
- Make sure the lighting in the room is adequate.

TEACHING PATIENTS WITH LEARNING DISABILITIES

Determine the type of learning disability in order to design teaching:

- When a patient has a **visual problem**, the nurse should use **verbal teaching**, repeated several times as needed and record the session for the patient to hear later if possible or use prepared audiotapes or CDs containing the information. The patient should verbalize learning to show attainment of the learning goal.
- When **auditory perception** is a problem, learning materials should be **visual** with as few words as possible. Demonstration, role-playing, and practicing the procedure will be useful to the patient. Printed materials should employ pictures, and computer use can be useful.
- If the patient has an **expressive problem**, he/she needs time to process the input and to ask questions. **Hand gestures, demonstrations, and the senses** should be utilized for teaching when appropriate.

A developmental disability will require information presented in a format that is appropriate for the person's developmental level. The nurse should keep explanations simple, and use gestures, demonstrations, activities, and repetition to teach.

TEACHING TO DISABLED PATIENTS AND FAMILIES

The teaching of disabled patients and their families begins with an assessment of the family's willingness and preparation for the heavy duty of care that will be required. The nurse must teach information about diseases or disabilities as well as medications, procedures, diet, and physical therapies. The patients must be taught to perform ADLs as well as possible and caregivers taught how to assist when needed:

- Give patients enough information to understand and manage the disabilities and to empower them with a sense of control and coping.
- Don't overwhelm them with information.
- Plan the teaching to provide information according to learning readiness and priorities but be flexible and change the plan if needed.
- Utilize checklists of skills to help keep track of all that has been learned.
- Give praise, continued feedback, support, and empathy with every teaching session.
- Provide resources that patients and family can use after discharge and refer to home health for continuing support and teaching.

IMPORTANCE OF PATIENT'S CULTURE IN DESIGN OF TEACHING PLAN

The nurse must always assess the individual's cultural beliefs and values and not assume that they are the same as the culture on a whole. These beliefs determine what information the patient feels that they can pursue. Teaching that conflicts with these beliefs will be rejected. The patient's perception of health and the healthcare system must be determined because a lack of confidence in the teacher can impair motivation to learn. The nurse must **assess the patient's beliefs** about the following to develop a personalized teaching plan:

- Body image, self-esteem
- Abilities and level of knowledge
- Principles of living
- Diet, activity, health practices
- Involvement of family and support persons
- Physical and mental health and disease
- Causes of disease
- Aging
- Gender issues
- Spirituality, customs, rituals, religious precepts

Care Coordination and Collaboration

SKILLS NEEDED FOR COLLABORATION

Nurses must learn the set of skills needed for **collaboration** in order to move nursing forward. Nurses must take an active role in gathering data for evidence-based practice to support nursing's role in health care, and they must share this information with other nurses and health professionals in order to plan staffing levels and to provide optimal care to patients. Increased and adequate staffing has consistently been shown to reduce adverse outcomes, but there is a well-documented shortage of nurses in the United States, and more than half currently work outside the hospital setting. Increased patient loads not only increase adverse outcomes but also increase job dissatisfaction and burnout. In order to manage the challenges facing nursing, nurses must develop the following skills needed for collaboration:

- Be willing to compromise
- Communicate clearly
- Identify specific challenges and problems
- Focus on the task
- Work with teams

COMMUNICATION SKILLS

Collaboration requires a number of communication skills that differ from those involved in communication between nurse and patient. These skills include:

- **Using an assertive approach**: It's important for the nurse to honestly express opinions and to state them clearly and with confidence, but the nurse must do so in a calm, non-threatening manner.
- **Making casual conversation**: It's easier to communicate with people with whom one has a personal connection. Asking open-ended questions, asking about others' work, or commenting on someone's contributions helps to establish a relationship. The time before meetings, during breaks, and after meetings presents an opportunity for this type of conversation.
- **Being competent in public speaking**: Collaboration requires that a nurse be comfortable speaking and presenting ideas to groups of people. Speaking and presenting ideas competently also helps the nurse to gain credibility. Public speaking is a skill that must be practiced.
- **Communicating in writing**: The written word remains a critical component of communication, and the nurse should be able to communicate clearly and grammatically.

COMMUNICATION AND HAND OFFS

The nurse is usually the primary staff member responsible for **external and internal hand off transitions of care**, and should ensure that communication is thorough and covers all essential information. The best method is to use a standardized format:

- **DRAW**: Diagnosis, recent changes, anticipated changes, and what to watch for.
- **I PASS the BATON**: Introduction, patient, assessment, situation, safety concerns, background, actions, timing, ownership, and next.
- **ANTICipate**: Administrative data, new clinical information, tasks, illness severity, contingency plans.
- **5 Rs**: Record, review, round together, relay to team, and receive feedback.

A reporting **form** or checklist may be utilized to ensure that no aspect is overlooked.

For external transitions, the nurse must ensure that the type of transport team and monitoring is appropriate for patient needs, and provide insight when determining the most appropriate mode of transportation: ground transfer for short distance, helicopter for medium to long distance, and fixed-wing aircraft for long distances.

SBAR TECHNIQUE

The **SBAR technique** is used to hand-off a patient from one caregiver to another to provide a systematic method so that important information is conveyed:

- **(S) Situation**: Overview of current situation and important issues
- **(B) Background**: Important history and issues leading to current situation
- **(A) Assessment**: Summary of important facts and condition
- **(R) Recommendation**: Actions needed

SHIFT REPORTING

Shift reporting should include bedside handoff when possible with oncoming staff members. The nurse handing off the patient should follow a specific format for handoff (such as I PASS the BATON) so that handoff is done in the same manner every time, as this reduces the chance of omitting important information. The shift report should include introduction of the oncoming staff to the patient, the triage category or acuity level of the patient, diagnosis (potential or confirmed), current status, laboratory and imaging (completed or pending) and results if available, and medications or treatments administered and pending. Any monitoring equipment (pulse oximetry, telemetry) should be examined. Any invasive treatments (Foley catheter, IV) should be discussed and equipment examined. The nurse should report any plans for admission, transfer, or discharge. It is essential that all staff be trained in shift reporting and the importance of consistency.

COLLABORATION BETWEEN NURSE AND PATIENT/FAMILY

One of the most important forms of **collaboration** is that between the nurse and the patient/family, but this type of collaboration is often overlooked. Nurses and others in the healthcare team must always remember that the point of collaboration is to improve patient care, and this means that the patient and patient's family must remain central to all planning. For example, including family in planning for a patient takes time initially, but sitting down and asking the patient and family, "What do you want?" and using the Synergy model to evaluate patient's (and family's) characteristics can provide valuable information that saves time in the long run and facilitates planning and expenditure of resources. Families, and even young children, often want to participate in care and planning and feel validated and more positive toward the medical system when they are included.

COLLABORATION WITH EXTERNAL AGENCIES

The nurse must initiate and facilitate collaboration with **external agencies** because many have direct impacts on patient care and needs:

- **Industry** can include other facilities sharing interests in patient care or pharmaceutical companies. It's important for nursing to have a dialog with drug companies about their products and how they are used in specific populations because many medications are prescribed to women, children, or the aged without validating studies for dose or efficacy.
- **Payers** have a vested interest in containing health care costs, so providing information and representing the interests of the patient is important.
- **Community groups** may provide resources for patients and families, both in terms of information and financial or other assistance.
- **Political agencies** are increasingly important as new laws are considered about nurse-patient ratios and infection control in many states.
- **Public health agencies** are partners in health care with other facilities and must be included, especially in issues related to communicable disease.

INTERDISCIPLINARY TEAMS

There are a number of skills that are needed to lead and facilitate coordination of **intra- and inter-disciplinary teams**:

- Communicating openly is essential. All members must be encouraged to participate as valued members of a cooperative team.
- Avoiding interrupting or interpreting the point another is trying to make allows free flow of ideas.
- Avoiding jumping to conclusions, which can effectively shut off communication.
- Active listening requires paying attention and asking questions for clarification rather than to challenge other's ideas.
- Respecting others' opinions and ideas, even when opposed to one's own, is absolutely essential.
- Reacting and responding to facts rather than feelings allows one to avoid angry confrontations and diffuse anger.
- Clarifying information or opinions stated can help avoid misunderstandings.
- Keeping unsolicited advice out of the conversation shows respect for others and allows them to solicit advice without feeling pressured.

LEADERSHIP STYLES

Leadership styles often influence the perception of leadership values and commitment to collaboration. There are a number of different **leadership styles**:

- **Charismatic**: Relies on personal charisma to influence people, and may be very persuasive, but this type leader may engage followers and relate to one group rather than the organization at large, limiting effectiveness.
- **Bureaucratic**: Follows organization rules exactly and expects everyone else to do so. This is most effective in handling cash flow or managing work in dangerous work environments. This type of leadership may engender respect but may not be conducive to change.
- **Autocratic**: Makes decisions independently and strictly enforces rules. Team members often feel left out of process and may not be supportive of the decisions that are made. This type of leadership is most effective in crisis situations, but may have difficulty gaining the commitment of staff.
- **Consultative**: Presents a decision and welcomes input and questions, although decisions rarely change. This type of leadership is most effective when gaining the support of staff is critical to the success of proposed changes.
- **Participatory**: Presents a potential decision and then makes final decision based on input from staff or teams. This type of leadership is time-consuming and may result in compromises that are not entirely satisfactory to management or staff, but this process is motivating to staff who feel their expertise is valued.
- **Democratic**: Presents a problem and asks staff or teams to arrive at a solution, although the leader usually makes the final decision. This type of leadership may delay decision-making, but staff and teams are often more committed to the solutions because of their input.
- **Laissez-faire ("free reign")**: Exerts little direct control but allows employees/teams to make decisions with little interference. This may be effective leadership if teams are highly skilled and motivated, but in many cases, this type of leadership is the product of poor management skills and little is accomplished because of this lack of leadership.

TEAM BUILDING

Leading, facilitating, and participating in performance improvement teams requires a thorough understanding of the dynamics of **team building**:

- **Initial interactions**: This is the time when members begin to define their roles and develop relationships, determining if they are comfortable in the group.
- **Power issues**: The members observe the leader and determine who controls the meeting and how control is exercised, beginning to form alliances.
- **Organizing**: Methods to achieve work are clarified and team members begin to work together, gaining respect for each other's contributions and working toward a common goal.
- **Team identification**: Interactions often become less formal as members develop rapport, and members are more willing to help and support each other to achieve goals.
- **Excellence**: This develops through a combination of good leadership, committed team members, clear goals, high standards, external recognition, spirit of collaboration, and a shared commitment to the process.

TEAM MEETINGS

Leading and facilitating improvement teams requires utilizing good **techniques for meetings**. Considerations include:

- **Scheduling**: Both the time and the place must be convenient and conducive to working together, so the leader must review the work schedules of those involved, finding the most convenient time. Venues or meeting rooms should allow for sitting in a circle or around a table to facilitate equal exchange of ideas. Any necessary technology, such as computers or overhead projectors, or other equipment, such as whiteboards, should be available.
- **Preparation**: The leader should prepare a detailed agenda that includes a list of items for discussion.
- **Conduction**: Each item of the agenda should be discussed, soliciting input from all group members. Tasks should be assigned to individual members based on their interest and part in the process in preparation for the next meeting. The leader should summarize input and begin a tentative future agenda.
- **Observation**: The leader should observe the interactions, including verbal and nonverbal communication, and respond to them.

COMMON VISION

Facilitating the creation of a common vision for care within the healthcare system begins with the organization/facility, working collaboratively to create teams and an organization focused on serving the patient/family. A common vision should be the ideal in any organization, but achieving such a goal requires a true collaborative effort:

- Inclusion of all levels of staff across the organization/facility, both those in nursing and non-nursing positions
- Consensus building through discussions, inservice, and team meetings to bring about convergence of diverse viewpoints
- Facilitation that values creativity and provides encouragement during the process
- Vision statement incorporating the common vision that is accessible to all staff
- Recognition that a common vision is an organic concept that may evolve over time and should be reevaluated regularly and changed as needed to reflect the needs of the organization, patients, families, and staff

FACILITATING CHANGE

Performance improvement processes cannot occur without organizational change, and **resistance to change** is common for many people, so coordinating collaborative processes requires anticipating resistance and taking steps to achieve cooperation. Resistance often relates to concerns about job loss, increased responsibilities, and general denial or lack of understanding and frustration. Leaders can prepare others involved in the process of change by taking these steps:

- Be honest, informative, and tactful, giving people thorough information about anticipated changes and how the changes will affect them, including positives.
- Be patient in allowing people the time they need to contemplate changes and express anger or disagreement.
- Be empathetic in listening carefully to the concerns of others.
- Encourage participation, allowing staff to propose methods of implementing change, so they feel some sense of ownership.
- Establish a climate in which all staff members are encouraged to identify the need for change on an ongoing basis.
- Present further ideas for change to management.

CONFLICT RESOLUTION

Conflict is an almost inevitable product of teamwork, and the leader must assume responsibility for **conflict resolution.** While conflicts can be disruptive, they can produce positive outcomes by opening dialogue and forcing team members to listen to different perspectives. The team should make a plan for dealing with conflict. The best time for conflict resolution is when differences emerge but before open conflict and hardening of positions occur. The leader must pay close attention to the people and problems involved, listen carefully, and reassure those involved that their points of view are understood. Steps to conflict resolution include:

- Allow both sides to present their side of conflict without bias, maintaining a focus on opinions rather than individuals.
- Encourage cooperation through negotiation and compromise.
- Maintain the focus, providing guidance to keep the discussions on track and avoid arguments.
- Evaluate the need for re-negotiation, formal resolution process, or third-party involvement.
- Utilize humor and empathy to diffuse escalating tensions.
- Summarize the issues, outlining key arguments.
- Avoid forcing resolution if possible.

HEALTHCARE TEAM MEMBERS

ROLE OF NURSING CARE TO SUPPORT THERAPIES PROVIDED BY OTHER DISCIPLINES

Nursing care often involves providing **support to therapies** provided by other disciplines. The nurse works as a team member with physicians, occupational and physical therapists, respiratory therapists, social workers, and discharge planners. Floor nurses may work with nurses in other specializations, such as critical care or psychiatric nurses. As a primary coordinator of the care plan, the nurse ensures that the necessary therapies from all disciplines are administered as ordered, and maintains clear communication with all members of the patient's healthcare team. Nurses also support nutritional services by assuring that the patient receives the proper diet for the particular medical or surgical condition, and they communicate with housekeeping to ensure that the patient's environment is appropriate.

OCCUPATIONAL THERAPY

The function of occupational therapy is to enable the patient to attain functional outcomes that enhance health, prevent further injury or impairment, and sustain or improve the highest attainable level of independence. The occupational therapist's role is to **facilitate interventions** that aid the patient in improving basic motor and cognitive skills and to **introduce strategies** for meeting challenges at work or at home. In cases of permanent disability or loss of mobility, the occupational therapist works with the patient on adaptive measures to improve function and the ability to perform daily living tasks. Occupational therapists may use physical exercises to improve muscle strength, balance, and dexterity, or cognitive exercises and strategies to improve problem-solving and memory. They help patients with disabilities or cognitive impairments adapt to particular environments, such as a private home or workplace, and teach patients how to use adaptive equipment like wheelchairs, orthotic devices, or computer programs.

RESPIRATORY THERAPY

The function of respiratory therapy is to provide care to patients with **respiratory and cardiopulmonary disorders**. The role of the respiratory therapist is to diagnose, evaluate, and treat patients with these disorders, and manage their therapeutic care. The respiratory therapist administers aerosolized medications and provides bronchopulmonary hygiene and postural drainage therapy. The role of the respiratory therapist is also to provide support for mechanically-ventilated patients and to maintain an artificial or natural airway. Many respiratory therapists perform pulmonary function testing as well as hemodynamic monitoring. Some respiratory therapists obtain arterial blood gases and other blood samples, as well as assemble and maintain respiratory equipment. They also teach patients how to self-administer aerosol medications and use life-support respiratory equipment in the home environment.

CASE MANAGER

The case manager is an RN that works for a healthcare insurer as a **manager of the provision of healthcare services** to the people the company insures. One manager or a group of managers are given a caseload of patients with the same range of diagnoses. The case manager is an expert in the range of diagnoses and coordinates services to fulfill the healthcare needs of that particular group of patients. The patient is followed throughout the continuum of care to ensure quality and cost-effectiveness of treatments and care. Complications are prevented and the incidence of repeat hospitalization is decreased. The case manager utilizes evidence-based pathways, clinical pathways, or other plans to track the care and progress of the patient. They are the ones who precertify care, negotiate for payment, and authorize treatment. Patient progress reports from the hospital utilization review or other liaison to the case manager are required at periodic intervals during the hospital stay.

IDENTIFYING THE NEED FOR PATIENT REFERRAL

Issues to consider when making patient referrals include:

- **Necessity**: The referral may be needed if the patient's needs are outside of the provider's scope or practice or field of expertise and if the provider cannot provide adequate assessment and treatment for the patient's condition.
- **Insurance requirements**: The provider should determine whether the patient's carrier requires preauthorization or other steps to make sure the patient's referral is covered.
- **Selection of specialist/therapist**: The specialist, in many cases, must be selected from a group of physicians who are participating in an insurance plan if the service is to be covered completely or at all by the insurance company. When possible, the patient should be given choice of referrals.
- **Submission**: The referral should be sent along with appropriate records and releases. The provider may need to make personal contact if specialists are selective, have waiting lists, and may not approve a referral.

FIVE RIGHTS OF DELEGATION

Prior to delegating tasks, the nurse should assess the needs of the patients and determine the task that needs to be completed, assure that he/she can remain accountable and can supervise the task appropriately, and evaluate effective completion. The **5 rights of delegation** include:

- **Right task**: The nurse should determine an appropriate task to delegate for a specific patient. This would not include tasks that require assessment or planning.
- **Right circumstance**: The nurse has considered the setting, resources, time factors, safety factors, and all other relevant information to determine the appropriateness of delegation. A task that is usually in one's scope (such as feeding a patient) may require assessment that makes it inappropriate to delegate (feeding a new stroke patient).
- **Right person**: The nurse is in the right position to choose the right person (by virtue of education/skills) to perform a task for the right patient.
- **Right direction**: The nurse provides a clear description of the task, the purpose, any limits, and expected outcomes.
- **Right supervision**: The nurse is able to supervise, intervene as needed, and evaluate performance of the task.

DELEGATION OF TASKS IN TEAMS

On major responsibility of leadership and management in performance improvement teams is using **delegation** effectively. The purpose of having a team is so that the work is shared, and leaders can cripple themselves by taking on too much of the workload. Additionally, failure to delegate shows an inherent distrust in team members. Delegation includes:

- Assessing the skills and available time of the team members, determining if a task is suitable for an individual
- Assigning tasks, with clear instructions that include explanation of objectives and expectations, including a timeline
- Ensuring that the tasks are completed properly and on time by monitoring progress but not micromanaging
- Reviewing the final results and recording outcomes

Because the leader is ultimately responsible for the delegated work, mentoring, monitoring, and providing feedback and intervention as necessary during this process is a necessary component of leadership. Even when delegated tasks are not completed successfully, they represent an opportunity for learning.

General Principles of Medication Administration

Principles of Pharmacology

PRINCIPLES OF PHARMACOKINETICS

Pharmacokinetics relates to the route of administration, the absorption, the dosage, the frequency of administration, the distribution, and the serum levels achieved over time.

- The **drug's rate of clearance (elimination)** and **doses needed** to ensure therapeutic benefit are considered. Most drugs are cleared through the kidneys, with water-soluble compounds excreted more readily than protein-soluble compounds.
- **Volume of distribution** (IV drug dose divided by plasma concentration) determines the rate at which the drug passes into tissue. Drug distribution depends on the degree of protein binding and ion trapping that takes place.
- **Elimination half-life** is the time needed for the concentration of a particular drug to decrease to half of its starting dose in the body. Approximately five half-lives are needed to achieve steady-state plasma concentrations if giving doses intermittently.
- **Context-sensitive half-life** is the time needed to reach 50% concentration after withdrawal of a continuously-administered drug.
- **Recovery time** is the length of time it takes for plasma levels to decrease to the point that the effect is eliminated. This is affected by plasma concentration.
- **Effect-site equilibrium** is the time between administration of a drug and clinical effect (the point at which the drug reaches the appropriate receptors) and must be considered when determining dose, time, and frequency of medications.
- The **bioavailability** of drugs may vary, depending upon the degree of metabolism that takes place before the drug reaches its site of action.

PRINCIPLES OF PHARMACODYNAMICS

Pharmacodynamics relates to biological effects (therapeutic or adverse) of drug administration over time. Drug transport, absorption, means of elimination, and half-life must all be considered when determining effects. Responses may include continuous responses, such as blood pressure variations, or dichotomous response in which an event either occurs or does not (such as death). Information from pharmacodynamics provides feedback to modify medication dosage (pharmacokinetics). Drugs provide biological effects primarily by interacting with receptor sites (specific protein molecules) in the cell membrane. Receptors include voltage-sensitive ion channels (sodium, chloride, potassium, and calcium channels), ligand-gated ion channels, and transmembrane receptors. Agonist drugs exert effects after binding with a receptor while antagonist drugs bind with a receptor but have no effects, so they can block agonists from binding. The total number of receptors may vary, upregulating or downregulating in response to stimuli (such as drug administration). Dose-response curves show the relationship between the amount of drug given and the resultant plasma concentration and biological effects.

FIRST PASS METABOLISM AND DRUG CLEARANCE

First pass metabolism is the phenomenon that occurs to ingested drugs that are absorbed through the gastrointestinal tract and enter the hepatic portal system. Drugs metabolized on the first pass travel to the liver, where they are broken down, some to the extent that only a small fraction of the

43

active drug circulates to the rest of the body. This first pass through the liver greatly reduces the bioavailability of some drugs. Routes of administration that avoid first pass metabolism include intravenous, intramuscular, and sublingual. **Drug clearance** refers to the ability to remove a drug from the body. The two main organs responsible for clearance are the liver and the kidneys. The liver eliminates drugs by metabolizing, or biotransforming the substance, or excreting the drug in the bile. The kidneys eliminate drugs by filtration or active excretion in the urine. Drugs use either renal or hepatic methods of clearance. Kidney and liver dysfunction inhibit the clearance of drugs that rely on that organ for removal. Toxicity results from poor clearance.

Enterohepatic Recirculation of Drugs and Renally-Excreted Drugs

Enterohepatic recirculation refers to the process whereby a drug is effectively removed from circulation and then reabsorbed. The drug is secreted in bile, which is collected in the gall bladder and emptied into the small intestine, from which part of it is reabsorbed and part excreted in the feces. This reabsorption reduces the clearance of these drugs and increases their duration of action. Generally, drugs susceptible to enterohepatic recirculation are those with a molecular weight greater than 300 g/mol and those that are amphipathic (have both a lipophilic portion and a polar portion).

Renally-excreted drugs are metabolized (biotransformed) by the liver to a form that can be excreted by the kidneys. Others are excreted by the kidneys unchanged. Infants with decreased renal function demonstrate decreased urine output or elevated levels of BUN and creatinine. The nurse should avoid using drugs that depend on the kidneys for clearance if the infant has renal impairment as overdose may result.

Absorption in Relation to Routes of Medication Administration

The absorption rate of a drug depends on its transfer from its site of administration to the circulatory system. Different **routes of administration** have different absorption characteristics:

- **Oral**: Ingested medications pass from the gastrointestinal tract into the blood stream. Most absorption occurs in the small intestine and is affected by gastric motility and emptying rate, drug solubility in gastrointestinal fluids, and food presence. Orally administered drugs are susceptible to first pass metabolism by the liver.
- **Intravenous**: Medications directly administered to the blood stream have 100% absorption. Peak serum levels are rapidly achieved. Some drugs are not tolerated intravenously, due to vein irritation or toxicity, and others must be given as an infusion.
- **Intramuscular**: Medications injected into a muscle are absorbed fairly rapidly because muscle tissue is highly vascularized. Drugs in lipid vehicles absorb more slowly than those in aqueous vehicles.
- **Subcutaneous**: Medications injected beneath the skin absorb more slowly because the dermis is less vascularized than muscle. Hypoperfusion and edema decrease absorption further.

Blood Drug Levels

Plasma drug levels are used for **therapeutic drug monitoring** because, although plasma is often not the site of action, plasma levels correlate well with therapeutic (effective) and toxic (dose-related adverse effects) responses to most drugs. The therapeutic range of a drug is that between the minimum effective concentration (level at which there is no therapeutic benefit) and the toxic concentration (level at which toxic effects occur). To achieve drug plateau (steady state), the drug half-life (time needed to decrease drug concentration by 50%) must be considered. Most drugs reach plateau with administration equal to four half-lives and completely eliminate a drug in 5 half-lives. Because drug levels fluctuate, peak (highest drug concentration) and trough (lowest drug concentration) levels may be monitored. Samples for trough levels are taken immediately prior to administration of another dose while peak samples are taken at various times, depending on the average peak time of the specific drug, which may vary from 30 minutes to 2 hours or so after administration.

SIDE EFFECTS OF MEDICATIONS

All drugs can have side effects, and some are toxic at certain levels or in combination with other drugs. Some side effects will be minor and may go away after a week or two. Others can be severe or life threatening, such as anaphylaxis. Common side effects include nausea, vomiting, diarrhea, and rashes. Side effects may vary with individuals according to age, gender, and condition and may be related to non-compliance with treatment, incorrect dosage, polypharmacy, or drug interactions. Drug compendiums will list all possible side effects according to system or incidence. Pharmacologically similar medications usually have some common side effects among the drugs in that class. Nursing actions include:

- Always question the patient about allergies or previous drug reactions before administering medication.
- Educate the patient about possible side effects of all medications.
- Watch out for drug/drug or food/drug combinations that are dangerous.

DRUG INTERACTIONS

Drug interactions occur when one drug interferes with the activity of another in either the pharmacodynamics or pharmacokinetics:

- With **pharmacodynamic interaction,** both drugs may interact at receptor sites causing a change that results in an adverse effect or that interferes with a positive effect.
- With **pharmacokinetic interaction**, the ability of the drug to be absorbed and cleared is altered, so there may be delayed effects, changes in effects, or toxicity. Interactions may include problems in a number of areas:
  - **Absorption** may be increased or (more commonly) decreased, usually related to the effects within the gastrointestinal system.
  - **Distribution** of drugs may be affected, often because of changes in protein binding.
  - **Metabolism** may be altered, often causing changes in drug concentration.
  - **Biotransformation** of the drug must take place, usually in the liver and gastrointestinal system, but drug interactions can impair this process.
  - **Clearance interactions** may interfere with the body's ability to eliminate a drug, usually resulting in increased concentration of the drug.

SPECIFIC INTERACTIONS

Some drugs will either increase or inhibit the actions of other drugs. They may interfere with receptor-site binding or the way in which the drug is metabolized or excreted. Certain drugs may cause drowsiness when taken together or with alcohol. Some foods will inhibit drug action, such as the inhibition of warfarin by vitamin K-containing foods. Other foods may cause toxic levels of a drug to accumulate. Grapefruit juice, for example, is metabolized by the same enzyme that metabolizes about 50 drugs, including digoxin and statins, and this can prevent the liver from breaking down drugs and lead to severe reactions. The nurse should always obtain a complete medication list from the patient, including prescription and over-the-counter medications, herbals, vitamins, minerals, and dietary supplements that are taken regularly and occasionally. All medications taken should be checked for **potential interactions with drugs or foods.**

Principles of Adult Medication Administration

DRUG CLASSIFICATION

The following are different ways to classify drugs:

- **Therapeutic classification**: The common uses for the drug will place it in a certain therapeutic classification.
- **Pharmacological classification**: The action of the drug determines which pharmacological category a drug will be in.

All drugs have a **chemical name** and a **generic name,** which is simpler. A company making the drug can give it a **trade or brand name**. The generic form of a drug is generally cheaper but may differ in efficacy from a brand name drug due to a difference in the amount of drug that is absorbed for use in the body. The Controlled Substances Act restricts usage of certain drugs and classifies them according to schedules that include:

- **Schedule I**: Ecstasy, LSD, marijuana, peyote, Quaalude®, mescaline, psilocybin, heroin, and others
- **Schedule II**: Amphetamine, cocaine, codeine, fentanyl, Dilaudid®, Demerol®, Ritalin®, morphine, opium, and others
- **Schedule III**: Anabolic steroids, barbiturates, codeine, Vicodin®, and pentothal
- **Schedule IV**: Xanax®, Librium®, Klonopin®, Tranxene®, Redux®, Darvocet®, Valium®, Ativan®, Equagesic®, Versed®, phenobarbital, Restoril®, Sonata®, Ambien®
- **Schedule V**: Lomotil® and others

5 RIGHTS OF MEDICATION ADMINISTRATION

The 5 rights of medication administration are used to prevent/reduce medication errors in the hospital setting. Often these 5 rights are integrated into the scanning requirements of electronic documentation. The **5 rights of medication administration** must also be incorporated into the prescriber's order:

- **Right Patient**: Confirm the patient's identity using two identifiers, often being their full name and date of birth. Scanning will also confirm the patient's identity with their bar code and electronic health record.
- **Right Drug**: Check the name of the drug with the prescriber's order. By scanning the medication, the drug name will also be checked against the order.
- **Right Dose**: Check the dose of the drug with the prescriber's order. Some medications require a second nurse confirm any dosage calculations utilized before administration. Ensure the dosage is appropriate and contact the prescriber if there are any concerns.
- **Right route**: Routes include oral (PO), subcutaneous, intradermal, IV, or IM, amongst others. The route must also be confirmed with the prescriber's order.
- **Right time/frequency**: The drug may be administered as a one-time dose, PRN (as needed), or recurring administration (twice daily, every 8 hours, etc.).

CLINICAL SITUATIONS THAT HAVE IMPLICATIONS FOR MEDICATION ADMINISTRATION

It is quite important to recognize clinical situations involving patients that may have **implications for the administration of medications**. For example, many patients have co-morbid conditions that will impact decisions about their medication administration. A patient with non-insulin-dependent diabetes and coronary artery disease who is being treated for a hip fracture would require oral hypoglycemic medications, cardiovascular medications, pain medication, and anticoagulants. Another example would be an insulin-dependent diabetic patient with concomitant hypertension and renal failure. This patient would require insulin, anti-hypertensive medications, and dosing adjustments of medications secondary to renal failure. The nurse who is responsible for the patient must ensure that the correct dosages of each prescribed medication are administered on time. Potential negative side effects and drug-drug interactions should be avoided, and the patient should be monitored for adverse reactions to newly prescribed drugs.

ROUTES OF DRUG ADMINISTRATION

The route of administration is the manner by which a drug is introduced into the body. The most **common routes of administration** are:

- Enteral (oral, rectal, or by feeding tube)
- Topical (on the skin, in the eyes or nose, vaginal, or inhaled)
- Parenteral (IV, subcutaneous, intramuscular, intracardiac, intraosseous, intradermal, intrathecal, intraperitoneal, transdermal, transmucosal, intravitreal, and epidural)

There are many variations on these three basic routes of administration. The FDA acknowledges 111 different routes of administration. When deciding on the route of administration, the doctor and pharmacist consider:

- How fast the patient requires the drug
- How effective it will be by a given route
- The likelihood of toxicity
- The discomfort it will cause
- How likely the patient is to comply with the route
- How likely the route is to play into the patient's addictive habits

INJECTIONS

The three most common types of injections and the preferred injection sites are as follows:

- **Subcutaneous Injection**: Deliver the drug under the skin with a ½ inch, 24- or 25-gauge needle held at a 45° angle to reach the fat. Choose the upper arm, abdomen, thigh, or lower back as the site. The maximum amount of subcutaneous medication is 0.5 ml. An example is insulin for a patient with diabetes.
- **Intramuscular Injection**: Deliver the drug into the muscle at a 90° angle to reach the deep tissue. Standard needle length is 1 to 1.5 inches depending on the weight of the individual. CDC guidelines recommend the use of a 22- to 25-gauge needle for adult intramuscular injections. Recommended sites for injection on the adult include deltoid (most recommended), vastus lateralis (thigh), ventrogluteal (hip), or dorsogluteal (buttocks). The maximum recommended amount of IM medication is 3 mL. An example is Vitamin B12 for a patient with pernicious anemia.
- **Intravenous Injection**: Deliver the drug into a vein of the arm, hand, leg, foot, scalp, or neck with an Angiocath, butterfly, or Insyte Autoguard needle. Use a size from 14 gauge to 26 gauge, depending on the fluid and the patient. The nurse sets the drip rate per minute by adjusting the clamp and monitoring the drip chamber. An example of a drug requiring intravenous injection is Zoledronate, which is given yearly to prevent bone fractures for individuals with osteoporosis.

> **Review Video: Calculating IV Drip Rates**
> Visit mometrix.com/academy and enter code: 396112

Two less frequently used forms of injection are: Intradermal (into the skin) for Mantoux TB test, and intraosseous access (IO) into the bone, which is used in emergency situations when other access sites are not available.

HERBAL-DRUG CONTRAINDICATIONS

Patients on certain medications should not take some herbals. Some **contraindications for common herbals** include:

- **Echinacea**: Anti-anxiety meds, antifungals, heart medications, HIV medications, anabolic steroids, methotrexate, NSAIDs
- **Gingko Biloba**: Anticoagulants, NSAIDs, aspirin, acetaminophen
- **Garlic**: Anticoagulants, oral hypoglycemics, NSAIDs
- **Licorice**: Diuretics, digoxin, antihypertensives
- **St. John's Wort**: Antidepressants, anticoagulants, Tamoxifen, oral contraceptives, HIV medications, anesthetics. Action is similar to MAO inhibitor
- **Valerian**: Sedatives, anti-seizure meds, anesthetics, alcohol, opioids
- **Feverfew**: Anticoagulants, migraine meds, NSAIDs
- **Ginger**: Anticoagulants, NSAIDs
- **Ginseng**: Anticoagulants, antihypertensives, NSAIDs, opioids. Do not take when pregnant or lactating
- **Goldenseal**: Antihypertensives, diabetic medications, meds for kidney diseases. Do not take when pregnant or lactating
- **Kava-kava**: Alcohol, anti-seizure meds, antidepressants, sedatives, anesthetics, antipsychotics, NSAIDS, opioids
- **Saw Palmetto**: Hormone therapy
- **Hawthorn**: Digoxin

Alternative, Complementary, and Non-Pharmacologic Interventions

COMPLEMENTARY THERAPY

Complementary therapies are often used, either alone or in conjunction with conventional medical treatment. These methods should be included if this is what the patient/family chooses, empowering the family to take control of their plan of care. Complementary therapies vary widely and most can easily be incorporated. The **National Center for Complementary and Alternative Medicine** recognizes the following:

- **Whole medical systems**: Chinese medicine (acupressure, acupuncture), naturopathic and homeopathic medicines, and Ayurveda
- **Mind-body medicine**: Prayer, artistic creation, music and dance therapy, biofeedback, focused relaxation, and visualization
- **Biological medicine**: Aromatherapy, herbs, plants, trees, vitamins and minerals, and dietary supplements
- **Manipulation**: Massage and spinal manipulation
- **Energy medicines**: Magnets, electric current, pulsed fields, Reiki, qi gong, and laying-on of the hands

PRECAUTIONS

The use of alternative and complementary therapies should be thoroughly discussed by patients and their physician. Patients should be encouraged to use therapies that are shown to have a beneficial, complementary effect on conventional medical treatment. These therapies include the use of massage, superficial stimulation, relaxation, distraction, hypnosis, and guided imagery.

- Encourage patients to practice the techniques until they are proficient in their use to give them a chance to prove their value.
- Teach the patient how the therapies work to encourage the patient to believe in them to contribute to the placebo effect.
- Caution the patient against abandoning current medical treatment.
- Inform the patient of the high cost of alternate therapies that can divert needed funds and result in little or no benefit.
- Provide the patient with resources in the form of books, pamphlets, and informative websites that prove the results of scientific research so that they can evaluate alternative therapies for themselves.

WHOLE MEDICAL SYSTEMS

Whole medical systems are different philosophies and methods of explaining and treating health and illness. Some systems include:

- **Homeopathic medicine**: This European system uses small amounts of diluted herbs and supplements to help the body to recover from disease by stimulating an immune response.
- **Naturopathic medicine**: This is a European system that uses various natural means (herbs, massage, acupuncture) to support the natural healing forces of the body.
- **Chinese medicine**: Centers on restoring the proper flow of life forces within the body to cure disease by using herbs, acupressure and acupuncture, and meditation.
- **Ayurveda**: This is an Indian system that tries to bring the spirit into harmony with the mind and body to treat disease via yoga, herbs, and massage.

ESSENTIAL OILS AND CUPPING

Essential oils (concentrated oils from plants) are either inhaled (aromatherapy) or diluted and applied to the skin. Essential oils are believed to reduce stress, aid sleep, improve dermatitis, and aid digestion. Commonly used essential oils include eucalyptus, lavender, lemon, peppermint, rosemary, rose, and tea tree. Oils may cause skin irritation when applied to the skin.

Cupping is an ancient practice still used in Southeast Asia and the Middle East to reduce pain, promote healing, and improve circulation. With dry cupping, cups are heated by placing something flammable (such as paper or herbs) inside the cup and setting it on fire to heat the cup, which is then immediately placed on the back along the meridians (generally on both sides of the spine) to form a vacuum that draws blood to the skin and causes circular bruises believed to heal that part of the body. Wet cupping includes leaving the heated cup in place for three minutes, removing it, making small cuts in the skin, and then applying suction cups again to withdraw blood. Cupping should be avoided in children under 4 and limited to short periods in older children.

ACUPUNCTURE

Alternative systems of medical practice include acupuncture, homeopathy, and naturopathy. **Acupuncture**, an ancient Oriental practice, uses stainless steel or copper needles inserted into superficial skin layers at points where energy or life force called *qi* is believed to occur. The needles are supposed to restore balance and the flow of *qi*. The NIH has recognized the effectiveness of acupuncture for certain side effects of other cancer treatments, such as nausea, vomiting, and pain. However, there is no documented scientific evidence to support the principles expounded. Acupuncturists are certified through either formal coursework or apprenticeships, and there is also board certification in this area for physicians. The needles used are classified as class II, which means they have manufacturing and labeling requirements.

HERBAL REMEDIES AND REGULATIONS

In the United States, most **herbal preparations** are classified as dietary supplements. That means that they are not subject to the same rigorous manufacturing, safety, efficacy, and control practices as pharmaceutical drugs. Herbal supplements are only governed by the Dietary Supplement and Health Education Act (DSHEA). As long as no specific disease treatment or curative claims are made, the supplement can be marketed without limitation and safety concerns must be pursued by the FDA after the fact. Nevertheless, some herbal remedies have been undergoing clinical trials in the U.S. to substantiate their health-enhancing or traditional/historical or international use claims. However, the focal point of these studies is still only on the effectiveness of the specific supplement. In Europe, there has been some movement toward greater regulation and licensing of herbal products, but not to the extent of formal drug regulations.

TOXICITIES ASSOCIATED WITH HERBAL REMEDIES

Use of herbal preparations has been associated with a variety of **toxicities**, primarily in categories such as cardiovascular problems, hypersensitivity reactions, disorientation, gastrointestinal problems, and liver malfunction. Because quality control measures are relatively lax for these remedies, contamination from infectious agents and toxic metals can potentially cause other side effects. Many of these herbal medicines **interact with conventional drugs**, thus altering their pharmacodynamics. For example, St. John's wort, which is primarily used for depressive disorders or as a sedative, interacts with a wide range of traditional pharmacologic agents and suppresses their levels in the bloodstream. Kava kava, made from dried roots of a type of pepper bush, is used as a sedative, but it also has been associated with hepatic failure and via interactions with several other drugs can actually induce a comatose state. Ginseng is an Asian remedy touted for its curative properties in a number of diseases. However, it can react with steroidal drugs and induce shaking and manic episodes. These are just a few examples of potential dangers.

NON-PHARMACEUTICAL PAIN RELIEF

Non-pharmaceutical methods to relieve pain that can be used exclusively or combined with medications include massage, heat, cold, electrical stimulation, distraction, relaxation, imagery, visualization, and music. Other **alternatives or adjuncts to pain medication** include hypnosis, magnets, acupuncture, acupressure, and therapeutic touch. Herbs, aromatherapy, reflexology, homeopathic medicine, and prayer may also be accepted by the patient. Any method that the patient feels may help that isn't harmful should be used to help get relief.

MIND-BODY MEDICINE FOR PAIN AND DISEASE

Mind-body medicine (prayer, artistic creation, music and dance, biofeedback, relaxation, and visualization) can help distract people from pain or other symptoms if they are able to concentrate on the method. This can result in the transfer of less painful stimuli to the brain by stimulating the **descending control system**. These methods work if the patient can use them to create alternate sensations in the brain, but will not work if the patient is unable to concentrate due to intense pain.

Relaxation that occurs as a result of using these methods helps to reduce muscular tension that can make pain worse and reduces fatigue caused by chronic pain. Relaxation has been proven to be the most helpful after surgery. Postoperative patients report a greater feeling of control over their pain and tend to request fewer opioids to control pain. Biofeedback can help patients to recognize the feelings of both tension and relaxation and provide a way to indicate their success in managing muscle tension.

USE OF VISUALIZATION

There are a number of methods used for **visualization** to reduce anxiety and promote healing. Some include audiotapes with guided imagery, such as self-hypnosis tapes, but the patient can be taught basic **techniques** that include:

- Sit or lie comfortably in a **quiet place** away from distractions.
- Concentrate on **breathing** while taking long slow breaths.
- **Close the eyes** to shut out distractions and create an image in the mind of the place or situation desired.
- Concentrate on that **image**, engaging as many senses as possible and imaging details.
- If the mind wanders, breathe deeply and **bring consciousness back** to the image or concentrate on breathing for a few moments and then return to the imagery.
- End with positive imagery.

Sometimes, patients are resistive at first or have a hard time maintaining focus, so **guiding** them through visualization for the first few times can be helpful.

STIMULATION OF THE SKIN TO REDUCE PAIN

Skin, muscles, fascia, tendons, and the cornea contain **nociceptors** that are nerve endings that respond to painful stimuli. Massage, transcutaneous electrical nerve stimulation (TENS), heat and cold provide stimulation to other nerves that transfer only sensation, not pain. These signals block some of the transfer of the nociceptor impulses:

- **Massage** not only sends alternate sensation to the brain, but also results in relaxation that decreases the muscular tension that contributes to pain.
- **TENS** works well on incisional and neuromuscular pain by providing a gentle electrical stimulation that overrides the painful impulses from the area and may stimulate endorphins.
- **Heat therapy** increases blood flow and oxygen to promote healing and stimulates neural receptors, decreasing pain. Heat also helps loosen tense muscles that may be contributing to pain.
- **Cold therapy** decreases circulation and reduces production of chemicals related to inflammation, thereby reducing pain.

TEMPERATURE-CONTROLLED THERAPIES
METHODS OF HEATING AND COOLING

There are a number of different ways to **heat** (thermotherapy) or **cool** (cryotherapy) for **healing**:

- **Conduction**: Conveyance of heat, cold, or electricity through direct contact with the skin, such as with hot baths, ice packs, and electrical stimulation.
- **Convection**: Indirect transmission of heat in a liquid or gas by circulation of heated particles, such as with whirlpools and paraffin soaks.
- **Conversion**: Heating that results from converting a form of energy into heat, such as with diathermy and ultrasound.
- **Evaporation**: Cooling caused by liquids that evaporate into gases on the skin with a resultant cooling effect, such as with perspiration or vapo-coolant sprays.
- **Radiation**: Heating that results from transfer of heat through light waves or rays, such as with infrared or ultraviolet light.

SHORTWAVE DIATHERMY

Shortwave diathermy uses radio waves (27.12 megahertz) to **increase the temperature in subcutaneous tissue** and is used along with passive and active range of motion exercises to **improve range** in painful conditions such as inflammation of the muscles, tendons, and bursae. The radio waves (eddy currents) are transmitted through a capacitor or inductor in a continuous or pulse waveform. Temperatures increase about 15 °C in fatty tissue and 4-6 °C in muscular tissue. Shortwave diathermy should not be used over any organs containing fluid, including the eyes, heart, head, or over pacemakers as the diathermy may disrupt the settings. Because this treatment may increase cardiac demand, it should be avoided in those with preexisting cardiac conditions and should not be used over malignancies. Additionally, it is contraindicated in areas of inflammation because heating the tissue increases inflammation. It cannot be used over prostheses as the metal may heat and damage tissue. Shortwave diathermy should avoid the epiphyses in children, as it may stimulate abnormal growth.

MICROWAVE DIATHERMY

Microwave diathermy is used similarly to shortwave diathermy but has a lower rate of heat increase and penetrance so it is used for muscles and joints near the surface rather than deep muscles, such as the hip. Heat is created by **electromagnetic radiation** (9.15-14.50 MHz) and raises temperature in fatty tissues by about 10-12 °C and in muscular tissue by 3-4 °C. **Treatment** is usually given for 15-30 minutes per session and is followed by range of motion exercises (passive and active) to increase flexibility. Contraindications are similar to those of shortwave diathermy in that this treatment should not be used where increase in temperature may be detrimental, such as over organs containing fluid, areas of inflammation, and epiphyses of children. Additionally, it should not be used over prostheses or pacemakers and should be avoided in those with cardiac disease.

SUPERFICIAL HEAT

Superficial heat with externally applied heat sources penetrates only the superficial layers of the skin (1-2 cm after about 30 minutes), but it is believed to relax deeper muscles by reflex, decrease pain, and increase metabolisms (2-3 times for every 10 °C increase in skin temperature). Therapeutic temperature range is 40-45 °C. **Superficial heat modalities** include:

- **Moist heat packs** placed on the skin and secured by several layers of towels to provide insulation, applied for 15-30 minutes.
- **Paraffin baths** (52-54 °C) with the hand, foot, or elbow dipped 7 times, cooling between dippings, and then wrapping with plastic and towels for 20 minutes.
- **Fluidotherapy** uses hot-air warmed (38.8-47.8 °C) cellulose particles into which a hand or foot is submerged for 20-30 minutes.

Passive and active range of motion exercises are done after superficial heat treatment. Contraindications include cardiac disease, peripheral vascular disease, malignant tumor, bleeding, and acute inflammation.

Deep heat differs from superficial heat in that the heat is generated internally using ultrasound, short wave, and microwave diathermy rather than applied to the surface of the skin. Deep heating has penetrance to 3-5 cm.

CRYOTHERAPY

Cryotherapy uses therapeutic cold treatment to cool the surface of the skin and underlying subcutaneous tissues in order to decrease blood flow, pain, and metabolism. Initially response to cold therapy causes **vasoconstriction** to occur within the first 15 minutes but if the tissues are cooled to -10 °C, then the body responds with **vasodilation**. Cryotherapy affects sensory response so the person will at first feel cold, which progresses to burning, aching, and finally to numbness and tingling. Treatment is usually given for 15-30 minutes. **Treatment modalities** include:

- **Ice packs** such as refrigerated gel packs (-5 °C) or plastic bags filled with water and ice chips are applied directly to the skin for 10-15 minutes for superficial cooling and 15-20 minutes for greater penetrance.
- A **towel dipped in ice and water slurry** is wrapped around limb to provide cold therapy, but this is best used only for emergency situations when ice packs are unavailable, as the towel must be changed frequently as the skin warms the towel rapidly.
- **Ice massage** is applied directly to the affected area for 5-10 minutes, usually rubbing the ice in circular motions on the skin surface. An ice massager is easily made by filled a paper cup with water and freezing it with a tongue depressor or Popsicle stick (to use as a handle) inserted into the center as the water starts to freeze. Then, the paper can be torn away from the bottom and sides when the ice is solid. Ice massage is often followed by friction massage.
- **Ice baths** (13-18 °C) are used for limbs, such as the lower leg, foot, or hand. The body part is immersed for 20 minutes.

Cryotherapy is usually followed by **active and passive exercises**. Contraindications include impaired circulation or sensation, cardiac disease, Raynaud's disease, and nerve trauma.

WHIRLPOOL BATHS

Whirlpool baths are used to increase **circulation** and promote **healing**. They are tubs with a turbine that mixes air with water, which is pressurized and flows into the tub water to create turbulence. Tubs are usually large enough to accommodate the full body although smaller limb-sized whirlpool tubs are available. Water temperature is 95-104 °F (adjusted for the individual) and should be deep enough to completely submerge the affected part. The body part should be cleaned with soap and water before immersion or a shower taken. If the full body is treated, then the patient should wear a swimming suit. During the whirlpool treatment, the muscles relax from the heat and **range of motion exercises** can be done while in the water. Typically, treatments last about 20 minutes, but the patient should be monitored, especially for the first 5 minutes, as some people become lightheaded and can lose consciousness.

CONTRAST BATHS

Contrast baths (alternating hot and cold) are used in the sub-acute phase of healing (after edema begins to subside) for **strains and sprains**. It is believed that contrast baths increase the circulation and help to further decrease edema by a pumping action as the **vasoconstriction and vasodilation** alternate. Two containers are filled with water, one with hot and the other with cold. The hot water should be maintained at about 100-110 °F and the cold at 55-65 °F. The cycle begins and ends with immersion in cold water. Cold water immersions usually last about 1 minute and hot water immersions 4 minutes. Typically, the affected limb is immersed in the cold water for 1 minute, removed, and immediately immersed in hot water for 4 minutes. This cycle is repeated about 3-4 times.

THERAPEUTIC ULTRASOUND

Ultrasound treats soft-tissue injuries (such as myositis, bursitis, and tendinitis) with sound waves (frequency 0.8-3 megahertz). Ultrasound utilizes a **piezoelectric crystal** that vibrates, producing sound waveforms, which are transmitted from the transducer through a gel substance into the tissue. The sound waves bounce off of the bone in an irregular pattern that causes an increase in temperature in the connective tissue, such as collagen fibers. Temperatures of the tissue may increase up to 43.5 °C, increasing metabolism in the area, neural conduction, as well as blood flow. Ultrasound is used to **decrease both contractures and scarring**. During treatment, the transducer passes in a circular motion about the skin surface, staying in contact with the gel medium. If a distal limb is submerged in water, the treatment is given with the head of the transducer 0.5-1 inch from the skin surface. Treatment is followed by range of motion exercises, passive and active. Contraindications are similar to other heat-producing modalities and include peripheral vascular disease, but ultrasound may be used over metal prostheses.

TENS

Transcutaneous electrical nerve stimulation (TENS) uses electrical stimulation to stimulate **peripheral sensory nerve fibers** to reduce acute or recurrent pain. TENS machines may be 2-lead or 4-lead and have adjustments for both frequency (1-20 Hz) and pulse width (50-300 microseconds, 10-50 mA). Stimulation can be intermittent or continuous. TENS units are small and battery-powered with wires and adhesive electrodes attached so that they can be worn while the person goes about usual activities. The positioning of the electrodes and the settings depend upon the site and type of injury, following guidelines provided by the manufacturer. The TENS machine can be used for a number of hours, but if used for days at a time, it will be less effective. TENS treatment is contraindicated with demand pacemakers and should not be used on the head or neck or over irritated skin.

REHABILITATION
SAID PRINCIPLE OF REHABILITATION AND RECONDITIONING

The Specific Adaptation to Imposed Demands (SAID) principle suggests that when a person is injured or stressed, that person attempts to overcome the problem by **adapting** to the demands of the situation. This is based on **Wolff's law** (systems adapt to demands). For example, if one hand is not usable, the person adapts and uses the other hand. Unfortunately, this adaptation can lead to increasing disability, so when the SAID principle is applied to rehabilitation, it means that the person must do exercises that specifically aim to correct the problem. Thus, the functional needs of the person should always be considered when designing a specific exercise program for that individual (such as treadmill running for soccer players). The exercise activities should as closely mirror the functional activities as possible. For example, if the goal is increased strength rather than endurance, then the exercise program should rely more heavily on strengthening exercises.

MASSAGE FOR REHABILITATION AND RECONDITIONING

Massage therapy is commonly used in sports and may be employed before activities, at breaks during activities, and after the activity is completed. Many types of massage are used in sports, and some massage therapists specialize in sports massage, but all nurses who work with athletes of any age should know the basic techniques of **sports massage** as it is used to both treat and prevent injuries. Sports massage is based primarily on Swedish massage although the massage may be deeper and targeted toward a particular injury, and other types of massage may be incorporated into a sports massage program. Massage of an injured area is delayed for the first **48-72 hours** to prevent further injury to tissues. Different techniques include:

- **Compression**: Deep rhythmical compressions of the muscles are done to increase circulation and temperature and make muscles more pliable. It may be used prior to deeper massage techniques.
- **Effleurage**: This is usually the beginning massage and begins softly and increases in intensity with the hands gliding over the tissue, so it is done with some type of oil or emollient. Massage is done in rhythmical broad strokes with the palms of the hands. This massage helps to relax the athlete and identify areas of tightness or pain that may require additional attention.
- **Friction**: These are massages either in line with muscle fibers or across the muscle fibers to create stretching and to reduce adhesions and scarring during healing. The tissue is pressed firmly against the underlying tissue and then pressure moves the underlying tissue until resistance is felt. Friction massage may be done deeply, and this can be uncomfortable. Usually, the thumb or fingers are used for this type of massage
- **Petrissage**: This is kneading massage and is usually used on large muscle areas, such as the calf or thigh. It increases circulation, so it is useful to relax and to improve circulation and drainage as well as to stretch muscles. The full hand is used for this massage with the heel and thumb stabilizing the tissue while the fingers squeeze the tissue.
- **Tapotement**: This type of massage uses quick rhythmic tapping, usually with the edge of the palm and little finger or the heel of the hand with the fingers elevated. It is done to increase circulation or relieve cramped muscles.
- **Vibration**: Vibratory massage is used for deep muscle relaxation and reduction of pain. Usually, the entire hand is placed against the skin, compressing the muscle and then vibrating the hand to cause movement.
- **Trigger point**: Pressure is applied with a finger or thumb to areas of point tenderness to reduce spasticity and pain.

55

PROGRESSION IN STRENGTHENING EXERCISES

Strengthening exercise progression includes the following exercises:

- **Isometric exercises** are done with the muscle and limb in static position with no movement of the joint or lengthening of the muscle. The muscle is contracted against resistance.
- **Isotonic exercises** include movement of the joint during exercise (such as running, weight lifting) and both shortening and lengthening of the muscles through eccentric or concentric contractions. Isotonic refers to tension, so the tension is constant during shortening and lengthening of the muscle.
- **Isokinetic exercises** utilize machines (such as stationary bicycles that can be set with various parameters) to control the rate and extent of contraction as well as the range of motion. Both speed and resistance can be set so the athlete is limited by the settings of the machine.
- **Plyometrics** is a particular type of exercise program that uses activities to allow a muscle to achieve maximal force as quickly as possible, and the sequence is a fast, eccentric movement (to stretch) followed quickly by a strong concentric movement (to contract).

Moral/Ethical/Legal Issues

Ethics

ETHICAL PRINCIPLES

Autonomy is the ethical principle that the individual has the right to make decisions about his or her own care. In the case of children or patients with dementia who cannot make autonomous decisions, parents or family members may serve as the legal decision maker. The nurse must keep the patient and/or family fully informed so that they can exercise their autonomy in informed decision-making.

Justice is the ethical principle that relates to the distribution of the limited resources of healthcare benefits to the members of society. These resources must be distributed fairly. This issue may arise if there is only one bed left and two sick patients. Justice comes into play in deciding which patient should stay and which should be transported or otherwise cared for. The decision should be made according to what is best or most just for the patients and not colored by personal bias.

Beneficence is an ethical principle that involves performing actions that are for the purpose of benefitting another person. In the care of a patient, any procedure or treatment should be done with the ultimate goal of benefitting the patient, and any actions that are not beneficial should be reconsidered. As conditions change, procedures need to be continually reevaluated to determine if they are still of benefit.

Nonmaleficence is an ethical principle that means healthcare workers should provide care in a manner that does not cause direct intentional harm to the patient:

- The actual act must be good or morally neutral.
- The intent must be only for a good effect.
- A bad effect cannot serve as the means to get to a good effect.
- A good effect must have more benefit than a bad effect has harm.

BIOETHICS

Bioethics is a branch of ethics that involves making sure that the medical treatment given is the most morally correct choice given the different options that might be available and the differences inherent in the varied levels of treatment. In the health care unit, if the patients, family members, and the staff are in agreement when it comes to values and decision-making, then no ethical dilemma exists; however, when there is a difference in value beliefs between the patients/family members and the staff, there is a bioethical dilemma that must be resolved. Sometimes, discussion and explanation can resolve differences, but at times the institution's ethics committee must be brought in to resolve the conflict. The primary goal of bioethics is to determine the most morally correct action using the set of circumstances given.

NURSING CODE OF ETHICS

There is more interest in the **ethics** involved in healthcare due to technological advances that have made the prolongation of life, organ transplants, prenatal manipulation, and saving of premature infants possible, sometimes with poor outcomes. Couple these with healthcare's limited resources, and **ethical dilemmas** abound. Ethics is the study of **morality** as the value that controls actions. The American Nurses Association Code of Ethics contains nine statements defining **principles** the nurse can use when faced with moral and ethical problems. Nurses must be knowledgeable about the many ethical issues in healthcare and about the field of ethics in general. The nurse must help a patient to reveal their values and morals to the health care team so that the patient, family, and team can resolve moral issues pertaining to the patient's care. As part of the healthcare team, the nurse has a right to express personal values and moral concerns about medical issues.

ETHICAL DECISION-MAKING MODEL

There are many ethical decision-making models. Some general guidelines to apply in using ethical decision-making models could be the following:

- Gather information about the identified problem
- State reasonable alternatives and solutions to the problem
- Utilize ethical resources (for example, clergy or ethics committees) to help determine the ethically important elements of each solution or alternative
- Suggest and attempt possible solutions
- Choose a solution to the problem

It is important to always consider the **ethical principles** of autonomy, beneficence, nonmaleficence, justice, and fidelity when attempting to facilitate ethical decision-making with family members, caregivers, and the healthcare team.

ETHICAL ASSESSMENT

While the terms *ethics* and *morals* are sometimes used interchangeably, ethics is a study of morals and encompasses concepts of right and wrong. When making **ethical assessments,** one must consider not only what people should do but also what they actually do, as these two things are sometimes at odds. Ethical issues can be difficult to assess because of personal bias, which is one of the reasons that sharing concerns with other internal sources and reaching consensus is so valuable. Issues of concern might include options for care, refusal of care, rights to privacy, adequate relief of suffering, and the right to self-determination. Internal sources might include the ethics committee, whose role is to make decisions regarding ethical issues. Risk management can provide guidance related to personal and institutional liability. External agencies might include government agencies, such as the public health department.

ETHICAL ANALYSIS OF A SITUATION

Assessment of the situation is done to reveal the **ethical, legal, and professional conflicts** that are present. Those who are involved are identified, including the patient, family, and healthcare personnel. The decision maker is determined if it is not the patient. Information about the situation is collected to determine medical facts about the disease and condition of the patient, options for treatment, and nursing diagnoses. Any pertinent legal information is included. The patient and family's cultural, religious, and moral values are determined. Possible courses of action are listed and compared in terms of outcomes for the patient using the utilitarian or deontological theory of ethics. Professional codes of ethics are also applied. A decision is made and evaluated as to whether it is the most morally correct action. Ethical arguments for and against the decision are given and responded to by the decision maker.

PROFESSIONAL BOUNDARIES
GIFTS

Over time, patients may develop a bond with nurses they trust and may feel grateful to the nurse for the care provided and want to express thanks, but the nurse must make sure to maintain professional boundaries. Patients often offer **gifts** to nurses to show their appreciation, but some adults, especially those who are weak and ill or have cognitive impairment, may be taken advantage of easily. Patients may offer valuables and may sometimes be easily manipulated into giving large sums of money. Small tokens of appreciation that can be shared with other staff, such as a box of chocolates, are usually acceptable (depending upon the policy of the institution), but almost any other gifts (jewelry, money, clothes) should be declined: "I'm sorry, that's so kind of you, but nurses are not allowed to accept gifts from patients." Declining may relieve the patient of the feeling of obligation.

SEXUAL RELATIONS

When the boundary between the role of the professional nurse and the vulnerability of the patient is breached, a boundary violation occurs. Because the nurse is in the position of authority, the responsibility to maintain the boundary rests with the nurse; however, the line separating them is a continuum and sometimes not easily defined. It is inappropriate for nurses to engage in **sexual relations** with patients, and if the sexual behavior is coerced or the patient is cognitively impaired, it is **illegal**. However, more common violations with adults, particularly elderly patients, include exposing a patient unnecessarily, using sexually demeaning gestures or language (including off-color jokes), harassment, or inappropriate touching. Touching should be used with care, such as touching a hand or shoulder. Hugging may be misconstrued.

ATTENTION

Nursing is a giving profession, but the nurse must temper giving with recognition of professional boundaries. Patients have many needs. As acts of kindness, nurses (especially those involved in home care) often give certain patients extra attention and may offer to do **favors**, such as cooking or shopping. They may become overly invested in the patients' lives. While this may benefit a patient in the short term, it can establish a relationship of increasing **dependency** and **obligation** that does not resolve the long-term needs of the patient. Making referrals to the appropriate agencies or collaborating with family to find ways to provide services is more effective. Becoming overly invested may be evident by the nurse showing favoritism or spending too much time with the patient while neglecting other duties. On the other end of the spectrum are nurses who are disinterested and fail to provide adequate attention to the patient's detriment. Lack of adequate attention may lead to outright neglect.

COERCION

Power issues are inherent in matters associated with professional boundaries. Physical abuse is both unprofessional and illegal, but behavior can easily border on abusive without the patient being physically injured. Nurses can easily **intimidate** older adults and sick patients into having procedures or treatments they do not want. Regardless of age, patients have the right to choose and the right to refuse treatment. Difficulties arise with cognitive impairment, and in that case, another responsible adult (often the patient's child or spouse) is designated to make decisions, but every effort should be made to gain patient cooperation. Forcing the patient to do something against his or her will borders on abuse and can sometimes degenerate into actual abuse if physical coercion is involved.

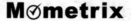

PERSONAL INFORMATION

When pre-existing personal or business relationships exist, other nurses should be assigned care of the patient whenever possible, but this may be difficult in small communities. However, the nurse should strive to maintain a professional role separate from the personal role and respect professional boundaries. The nurse must respect and maintain the confidentiality of the patient and family members, but the nurse must also be very careful about **disclosing personal information** about him or herself because this establishes a social relationship that interferes with the professional role of the nurse and the boundary between the patient and the nurse. The nurse and patient should never share secrets. When the nurse divulges personal information, he or she may become vulnerable to the patient, a reversal of roles.

Legal Regulations

ADVANCE DIRECTIVES

In accordance to Federal and state laws, individuals have the right to self-determination in health care, including the right to make decisions about end of life care through **advance directives** such as living wills and the right to assign a surrogate person to make decisions through a durable power of attorney. Patients should routinely be questioned about an advanced directive as they may present at a healthcare provider without the document. Patients who have indicated that they desire a do-not-resuscitate (DNR) order should not receive resuscitative treatments for terminal illness or conditions in which meaningful recovery cannot occur. Patients and families of those with terminal illnesses should be questioned as to whether the patients are Hospice patients. For those with DNR requests or those withdrawing life support, staff should provide the patient palliative rather than curative measures, such as pain control and/or oxygen, and emotional support to the patient and family. Religious traditions and beliefs about death should be treated with respect.

REGULATION OF NURSING BY STATES' NURSE PRACTICE ACT

Each state's **nurse practice act** seeks to regulate nursing within the state. It specifies the amount and type of education required to become an RN or LPN/LVN. It defines the nurse's role and responsibilities in healthcare settings. It lists actions that the nurse may take and defines advanced practice education, experience, responsibilities, and limitations. It gives nurses the authorization to perform as required. It also regulates delegation and supervision responsibilities of the nurse. Nurse practice acts are administered by the state board of nursing, which is responsible for issuing and renewing nurse licenses as well as discipline and censure of nurses. Most state boards of nursing now have a website that provides state-specific information about licensure and nursing rights and responsibilities.

NURSE'S ACCOUNTABILITY FOR NURSING CARE

Nurses are part of an interdisciplinary team responsible for patient outcomes. Nurses have the responsibility for the outcomes of nursing care as a professional group. This responsibility is outlined in each state's nurse practice act, the American Nurses Association (ANA) practice guidelines, and the nurse's job description. Tools, such as the nursing care plan that includes standardized nursing diagnoses, interventions, and expected outcomes, enable the nurse to fulfill this responsibility. Empowerment to act as the patient advocate allows the nurse to point out factors in the patient's individual situation that can be addressed to further improve outcome. Critical thinking during decision-making and detailed documentation are also important. The nurse is held accountable for delegation as well as supervising care by others and evaluation of the outcomes of that care as well. The nurse has personal **accountability** in terms of ethical and moral conduct. Since clinical knowledge is crucial to critical thinking, the nurse must strive to increase knowledge continuously through professional development throughout his or her career.

HIPAA

The Health Insurance Portability and Accountability Act (HIPAA) and state laws govern **who may receive healthcare information** about a person, how permission is to be obtained, how the information may be shared, and patients' rights concerning personal information. HIPAA strives to protect the **privacy** of an individual's healthcare information. Facilities must prevent this information from being accessed by unauthorized personnel. Healthcare information is required to be protected on the **administrative**, **physical**, and **technical** levels. The patient must sign a release form to allow any sharing of patient information. There are stiff penalties for violation of these laws, ranging from $100 for an unintentional violation to $50,000 for a willful violation. Facilities that violate HIPAA may also be subject to corrective actions. Penalties are governed by the Department of Health and Human Services' Office for Civil Right and the state attorneys general.

APPLICATION OF HIPAA TO PRACTICE

As an integral member of the health care team, the nurse must always be aware of HIPAA regulations and apply this knowledge to practice. The nurse is responsible for the following efforts to protect and maintain patient privacy:

- The nurse must read and follow facility policies regarding the transfer of patient data.
- Communication between health care personnel about a patient should always be in a private place so that this information is not overheard by those who do not have the right to share the information.
- Access to charts must be restricted to only those health care team members involved in that patient's care.
- Patient care information for unlicensed workers cannot be posted at the bedside, but must be on a care plan or the patient chart in a protected area.
- The nurse must not give information casually to anyone (e.g., visitors or family members) unless it is confirmed that they have the right to have that information.
- Family members must not be relied upon to interpret for the patient; an interpreter must be obtained to protect patient privacy.
- Computers with patient information must have passwords and safeguards to prevent unauthorized access of patient information.
- The nurse should not leave voicemail messages containing protected healthcare information for a patient but should instead ask the patient to call back.

> **Review Video: What is HIPAA?**
> Visit mometrix.com/academy and enter code: 412009

OSHA

The **Occupational Safety and Health Act (OSHA)** seeks to keep workers safe and healthy while on the job. OSHA mandates that employers maintain a safe environment, workers are made fully aware of any hazards, and that access to personal protective gear is made available to workers who come into contact with hazardous materials. By following these regulations, an employer keeps injury and illness of workers to an absolute minimum. This fosters productivity, since workers are not absent due to illness or injury, employee health costs are contained, and the turnover rate is decreased, saving money spent on hiring and training new employees. OSHA is concerned about healthcare employee exposure to radiation, as well as chemical and biological agents, when caring for patients. Information is available to help hospitals and other facilities write plans that comply with best practices to deal with this and other threats to employees. Cleaning procedures, decontamination, and hazardous waste disposal are all covered by OSHA and apply to everyday hospital operation as well as disaster situations.

> **Review Video: What is OSHA (Occupational Safety and Health Administration)**
> Visit mometrix.com/academy and enter code: 913559

AHRQ

The **Agency for Healthcare Research and Quality (AHRQ)** is part of the U.S. Department of Health and Human Services. This agency is concerned about health care and primarily promotes scientific research into the safety, effectiveness, and quality of healthcare. It encourages evidence-based healthcare that produces the best possible outcome while containing healthcare costs. It makes contracts with institutions to review any published evidence on healthcare in order to produce reports used by other organizations to write guidelines. The agency operates the National Guideline Clearinghouse, which is available online. It is a repository of evidence-based guidelines that address various health conditions and diseases. These guidelines are written by many different health-related professional organizations and are used by primary healthcare providers, nurses, and healthcare facilities to guide patient treatment and care.

OBRA 1987

The **Omnibus Budget Reconciliation Act of 1987 (OBRA 1987)**, also known as the Nursing Home Reform Act, instituted requirements for nursing homes with the purpose of strengthening and protecting patient rights. These requirements are as follows: "a facility must provide each patient with a level of care that enables him or her to attain or maintain the highest practicable physical, mental, and psychosocial wellbeing." OBRA 1987 required that all nursing home patients receive an initial evaluation with yearly follow-ups. Every patient is required to have a comprehensive care plan. Patients were ensured the right to medical care and the right to be informed about and refuse medical treatment. OBRA 1987 requires each state to establish, monitor, and enforce its own licensing requirements in addition to federal standards. Each state is also required to fund, staff, and maintain investigative and Ombudsman units.

OBRA 1990 (PSDA)

The Omnibus Budget Reconciliation Act of 1990 included the amendment called the **Patient Self Determination Act (PSDA)**. The PSDA required healthcare facilities to provide written information about advanced healthcare directives and the right to accept or reject medical or surgical treatments to all patients. Patients who make an advanced directive are leaving instructions about what medical interventions they authorize or refuse if they are incapacitated by illness or injury. They can also nominate another person to make these decisions for them in this situation. The PSDA also protected the right of patients to accept or refuse medical treatments. Healthcare facilities and hospitals are legally required to communicate these rights to all patients, to respect these rights, and to educate staff and personnel about these rights.

EMTALA

The **Emergency Medical Treatment and Active Labor Act (EMTALA)** is designed to prevent patient "dumping" from emergency departments (ED) and is an issue of concern for risk management that requires staff training for compliance:

- Transfers from the ED may be intrahospital or to another facility.
- Stabilization of the patient with emergency conditions or active labor must be done in the ED prior to transfer, and initial screening must be given prior to inquiring about insurance or ability to pay.
- Stabilization requires treatment for emergency conditions and reasonable belief that, although the emergency condition may not be completely resolved, the patient's condition will not deteriorate during transfer.
- Women in the ED in active labor should deliver both the child and placenta before transfer.
- The receiving department or facility should be capable of treating the patient and dealing with complications that might occur.
- Transfer to another facility is indicated if the patient requires specialized services not available intrahospital, such as to burn centers.

CMS

The **Centers for Medicare and Medicaid (CMS)**, part of the U.S. Department of Health and Human Service department, see to it that healthcare regulations are observed by healthcare facilities that receive federal reimbursement. They reimburse facilities for care given to Medicare, Medicaid, and the state Children's Health Insurance Program (CHIP) recipients. They also monitor adherence to HIPAA regulations concerning healthcare information portability and confidentiality. CMS examines documentation of patient care when deciding to reimburse for care given. CMS has regulations for all types of medical facilities, and these regulations have profoundly impacted nursing practice because nurses must ensure that they comply with regulations related to the quality of patient care and concerns regarding cost-containment. Each facility should provide guidelines to assist nursing staff in meeting the specific documentation requirements of CMS.

Patient Rights

PATIENT RIGHTS AND RESPONSIBILITIES

Empowering patients and families to act as their own advocates requires that they have a clear understanding of their **rights and responsibilities.** These should be given (in print form) and/or presented (audio/video) to patients and families on admission or as soon as possible:

- **Rights** include competent, non-discriminatory medical care that respects privacy and allows participation in decisions about care and the right to refuse care. They should have clear understandable explanations of treatments, options, and conditions, including outcomes. They should be apprised of transfers, changes in care plan, and advance directives. They should have access to medical records and billing information.
- **Responsibilities** include providing honest and thorough information about health issues and medical history. They should ask for clarification if they don't understand information that is provided to them, and they should follow the plan of care that is outlined or explain why that is not possible. They should treat staff and other patients with respect.

INFORMED CONSENT

The patient or their legal guardian must provide informed consent for all treatment the patient receives. This includes a thorough explanation of all procedures and treatment and associated risks. Patients/guardians should be apprised of all options and allowed to have input on the decision-making process. They should be apprised of all reasonable risks and any complications that might be life threatening or increase morbidity. The American Medical Association has established **guidelines for obtaining informed consent:**

- Explanation of the diagnosis
- Nature and reason for the treatment or procedure
- Risks and benefits of the treatment or procedure
- Alternative options (regardless of cost or insurance coverage)
- Risks and benefits of alternative options, including no treatment

Obtaining informed consent is a requirement in all states; however, a patient may waive their right to informed consent. If this is the case, the nurse should document the patient's waiving of this right and proceed with the procedure. Informed consent is not necessary for procedures performed to save life or limb in which the patient or guardian is unable to consent.

CONFIDENTIALITY

Confidentiality is the obligation that is present in a professional-patient relationship. Nurses are under an obligation to protect the information they possess concerning the patient and family. Care should be taken to safeguard that information and provide the privacy that the family deserves. This is accomplished through the use of required passwords when family call for information about the patient and through the limitation of who is allowed to visit. There may be times when confidentiality must be broken to save the life of a patient, but those circumstances are rare. The nurse must make all efforts to safeguard patient records and identification. Computerized record keeping should be done in such a way that the screen is not visible to others, and paper records must be secured.

Quality Improvement and Risk Assessment

CONTINUOUS QUALITY IMPROVEMENT

Continuous quality improvement is a multidisciplinary management philosophy that can be applied to all aspects of an organization, whether related to such varied areas as the cardiac unit, purchasing, or human resources. The skills used for epidemiologic research (data collection, analysis, outcomes, action plans) are all applicable to the analysis of multiple types of events, because they are based on solid scientific methods. Multi-disciplinary planning can bring valuable insights from various perspectives, and strategies used in one context can often be applied to another. All staff, from housekeeping to supervising, must be alert to not only problems but also opportunities for improvement. Increasingly, departments must be concerned with cost-effectiveness as the costs of medical care continue to rise, so the quality professional in the cardiovascular unit is not in an isolated position in an institution but is just one part of the whole, facing similar concerns as those in other disciplines. Disciplines are often interrelated in their functions.

JURAN'S QUALITY IMPROVEMENT PROCESS

Joseph Juran's quality improvement process (QIP) is a 4-step method of change (focusing on quality control) which is based on a trilogy of concepts that includes quality planning, control, and improvement. The steps to the QIP process include the following:

1. **Defining** the project and organizing includes listing and prioritizing problems and identifying a team.
2. **Diagnosing** includes analyzing problems and then formulating theories related to cause by root cause analysis and test theories.
3. **Remediating** includes considering various alternative solutions and then designing and implementing specific solutions and controls while addressing institutional resistance to change. As causes of problems are identified and remediation instituted to remove the problems, the processes should improve.
4. **Holding** involves evaluating performance and monitoring the control system in order to maintain gains.

FOCUS PERFORMANCE IMPROVEMENT MODEL

Find, organize, clarify, uncover, start (FOCUS) is a performance improvement model used to facilitate change:

1. **Find**: Identifying a problem by looking at the organization and attempting to determine what isn't working well or what is wrong.
2. **Organize**: Identifying those people who have an understanding of the problem or process and creating a team to work on improving performance.
3. **Clarify**: Determining what is involved in solving the problem by utilizing brainstorming techniques, such as the Ishikawa diagram.
4. **Uncover**: Analyzing the situation to determine the reason the problem has arisen or that a process is unsuccessful.
5. **Start**: Determining where to begin in the change process.

FOCUS, by itself, is an incomplete process and is primarily used as a means to identify a problem rather than a means to find the solution. FOCUS is usually combined with PDCA (FOCUS-PDCA), so it becomes a 9-step process; however, beginning with FOCUS helps to narrow the focus, resulting in better outcomes.

Nurse's Involvement in Quality Improvement

The following are ways in which nurses can be involved in quality improvement in their facility:

- **Identify situations** in the nursing unit that require improvement and might benefit patient outcomes (cost containment, incident reporting, etc.) if changed.
- **Identify potential items** that can be measured to be able to test the problem or to be able to monitor patient outcomes.
- **Collect data** on those measurements and determine current patient outcomes.
- **Analyze the data** and identify procedures, methods, etc., that can be utilized to potentially make positive changes in patient outcomes, doing research if necessary.
- **Make recommendations for changes** to be implemented to determine the effect on patient outcomes.
- **Implement recommendations** after approval from administrative personnel.
- **Collect data** using the same measurements and determine if the changes improved patient outcomes or not.

Risk Management

Risk management attempts to prevent harm and legal liability by being proactive and by identifying a patient's **risk factors**. The patient is educated about these factors and ways that they can modify their behavior to decrease their risk. Treatments and interventions must be considered in terms of risk to the patient, and the patient must always know these risks in order to make healthcare decisions. Much can be done to avoid mistakes that put patients at risk. Patients should note medications and other aspects of their care so that they can help prevent mistakes. They should feel free to question care and to have their concerns heard and addressed. When mistakes are made, the actions taken to remedy the situation are very important. The physician should be made aware of the error immediately, and the patient notified according to hospital policy. Errors must be evaluated to determine how the process failed. Honesty and caring can help mitigate many errors.

Nursing Malpractice, Negligence, Unintentional Torts, and Intentional Torts

- **Malpractice** is unethical or improper actions or lack of proper action by the nurse that may or may not be related to a lack of skills that nurses should possess.
- **Negligence** is the failure to act as any other diligent nurse would have acted in the same situation.
- Negligence can lead to an **unintentional tort**. In this case, the patient must prove that the nurse had a duty to act, a duty proven via standards of care, and that the nurse failed in this duty and harm occurred to the patient as a result of this failure.
- **Intentional torts** differ in that the duty is assumed and the nurse breached this duty via assault and battery, invasion of privacy, slander, or false imprisonment of the patient.

Foundations of Nursing Practice Test

Want to take this practice test in an online interactive format?
Check out the bonus page, which includes interactive practice questions and
much more: **https://www.mometrix.com/bonus948/nurseaceifn**

SCAN HERE

1. If a patient has been diagnosed with early osteoporosis, which of the following lifestyle changes may be most important?
    a. Weight loss
    b. High protein diet
    c. Smoking cessation
    d. Decreasing stress

2. Which of the following is the first-line drug for the relief of discomfort associated with osteoarthritis?
    a. NSAIDS (ibuprofen, naproxen)
    b. Acetaminophen (Tylenol®)
    c. Selective COX-2 inhibitors (celecoxib)
    d. Corticosteroids (prednisone)

3. When administering a tube feeding per a PEG tube, in what position should the nurse place the patient?
    a. Supine, flat
    b. Low Fowler's, 20°
    c. Semi-Fowler's, 45°
    d. High Fowler's, 90°

4. If a stroke patient has difficulty dressing himself or carrying out activities of daily living, which of the following therapies is most indicated?
    a. Occupational therapy
    b. Physical therapy
    c. Recreational therapy
    d. Mindfulness therapy

5. If a patient with a spinal cord injury exhibits signs of autonomic dysreflexia, what position should the patient be placed in?
    a. Trendelenburg
    b. Flat
    c. Low Fowler's
    d. High Fowler's

6. If a patient is hospitalized with kidney stones, what does the nurse anticipate doing?

   a. Maintaining contact precautions
   b. Limiting fluid intake
   c. Straining urine
   d. Catheterizing patient

7. Which of the following is generally the underlying cause of respiratory alkalosis?

   a. Hypoventilation
   b. Hyperventilation
   c. Elevated fever
   d. Dehydration

8. If a patient is prescribed short-term oxygen at 3 L per minute, what oxygen delivery device is most appropriate?

   a. Nasal cannula
   b. Face mask
   c. Oxygen conserving cannula
   d. Non-rebreather mask

9. What hemoglobin A1c level is recommended by the American Diabetes Association for most patients with diabetes mellitus type 2?

   a. 5%
   b. 6%
   c. 7%
   d. 8%

10. What oxygen saturation level indicates hypoxemia?

   a. <96%
   b. <94%
   c. <92%
   d. <90%

11. If a patient who receives chemotherapy has severe side effects, but the medication is justified because it provides more good than it does harm, this supports which of the following ethical principles?

   a. Justice
   b. Beneficence
   c. Nonmaleficence
   d. Veracity

12. Which of the following is a normal change associated with aging?

   a. Cognitive impairment
   b. Increased excretion of urine at night
   c. Anemia
   d. Heart disease

13. If an adolescent patient is angry at his doctor because he dislikes his treatment but insists the doctor is angry at him, what type of defense mechanism is the patient exhibiting?

    a. Projection
    b. Displacement
    c. Devaluation
    d. Dissociation

14. Which of the following is an example of secondary prevention?

    a. BP screening
    b. Fitness program
    c. Immunizations
    d. Cardiac rehabilitation program

15. If an older patient states that she sleeps only 3-4 hours each night, what should the next question be?

    a. "Why do you think that is?"
    b. "Do you drink caffeinated beverages in the evening?"
    c. "Are you confused during the night?'
    d. "Do you nap during the daytime or evening?"

16. Which of the following best describes the lesions associated with ulcerative colitis?

    a. Patchy lesions in the large and small intestines
    b. Continuous circumferential lesions in the rectum and colon
    c. Continuous lesions in the upper GI tract
    d. Patchy lesions in the rectum and colon

17. What is the first step in the nursing process?

    a. Evaluate
    b. Plan
    c. Assess
    d. Diagnose

18. If a patient has an ileostomy, what is the normal consistency of the stool?

    a. Liquid
    b. Watery, clear
    c. Mushy
    d. Formed

19. How many times a week should normal bowel movements occur?

    a. At least one time
    b. At least two times
    c. At least four times
    d. At least five times

20. If a patient is scheduled for a right-sided thoracentesis but is unable to sit up, how should the patient be positioned?

    a. Sidelying on the left side with the bed elevated 45°
    b. Sidelying on the left side with the bed flat
    c. Sidelying on the right side with the bed elevated 45°
    d. Prone with the bed flat

21. If a patient complains of abdominal pain, which of the following is the first thing to assess?

    a. Precipitating factors
    b. Severity of pain
    c. Frequency of pain
    d. Nature of pain

22. Which of the following increases the risk of hypokalemia?

    a. Chemotherapy
    b. Decreased urinary output
    c. Diarrhea and vomiting
    d. Traumatic injury

23. If a patient leaks urine when she coughs and when she feels the urge to urinate, this indicates what type of urinary incontinence?

    a. Stress
    b. Urge
    c. Functional
    d. Mixed

24. Which of the following is often the first sign of a urinary infection in an older adult with Alzheimer's disease?

    a. Sudden onset of increased confusion
    b. Pain
    c. Burning on urination
    d. Fever

25. If an older patient exhibits a sudden change in consciousness, including fluctuating confusion, hallucinations, and disorientation, the nurse should suspect which of the following?

    a. Dementia
    b. Delirium
    c. Bipolar disease
    d. Infection

26. Which of the following religious groups is likely to refuse blood transfusions because of religious beliefs?

    a. Buddhists
    b. Seventh Day Adventists
    c. Latter Day Saints (Mormons)
    d. Jehovah's Witnesses

27. What is the correct procedure for replacing soiled tracheostomy ties?

a. Remove soiled ties, hold tube in place, apply new ties
b. Remove soiled ties, secure tube with tape, apply new ties, remove tape
c. Apply new ties, remove soiled ties
d. Secure tube with tape, remove soiled ties, apply new ties

28. Which of the following are primary risk factors for the development of diabetes mellitus, type 2?

a. Poor nutrition and obesity
b. Older age and lack of exercise
c. Alcohol abuse
d. Use of alcohol and tobacco

29. If a patient dying of pancreatic cancer take high doses of an opioid to control pain, what is the primary concern?

a. The patient will become addicted
b. The patient will develop tolerance
c. The patient will develop bowel obstruction
d. The patient will overdose

30. Typically, how long should a patient avoid solid foods before an anesthetic?

a. 24 hours
b. 12 hours
c. 8 hours
d. 4 hours

31. Which finding is of most concern in the postoperative period when an adult patient is admitted to the recovery area?

a. Temperature 36 °C
b. Pulse 90 bpm
c. Oxygen saturation 96%
d. BP 80/46

32. If, during the postoperative period for abdominal surgery, the patient develops pain and slight redness and swelling in the right calf, this most likely indicates which of the following?

a. Muscle strain
b. Infection
c. Deep vein thrombosis
d. Trauma

33. Which of the following nursing interventions may help a patient reduce stress?

a. Reassure the patient that everything will be all right
b. Teach the patient to do deep breathing and relaxation exercises
c. Teach the patient about the causes of stress
d. Ask the patient about what is causing the stress

34. Which of the following nutritional elements is most necessary for the development and maintenance of bones and teeth?

  a. Calcium
  b. Magnesium
  c. Iron
  d. Sodium

35. If the nurse finds an older Asian patient trying to climb onto a toilet seat to get into a squatting position, what is the best response?

  a. Explain that the patient must sit on the toilet
  b. Assist the patient to squat on the toilet seat
  c. Provide a stool that elevates the patient's feet
  d. Ask the patient why she is trying to squat

36. If a patient is unable to move or turn independently, the patient is especially at risk for which of the following?

  a. Pressure sore
  b. Skin rash
  c. Muscle pain
  d. Infection

37. If the nurse finds a patient crying after the patient receives bad news, what is the most appropriate response?

  a. Ask the patient, "Why are you crying?"
  b. Say, "I'm so sorry you are upset."
  c. Leave the room and allow the patient privacy
  d. Say, "Try not to worry."

38. If a patient is using a standard walker after a stroke that resulted in left sided weakness, how should the patient use the walker?

  a. Move the walker ahead by 6 inches and then move the right leg forward followed by the left leg
  b. Move the walker ahead by 6 inches and then move the left leg forward followed by the right leg
  c. Move the walker and right leg ahead by 6 inches and then move the left leg
  d. Move the walker and left leg ahead by 6 inches and then move the right leg

39. Which of the following types of patients should be assessed for fall risk?

  a. Patients over 65
  b. Young children
  c. All patients
  d. Patients with confusion

40. If the body is properly aligned and balanced while standing, how should the toes point?

  a. Forward
  b. Laterally
  c. Slightly inward
  d. One forward and one laterally

41. How much time each week should an adult spend doing moderate intensity aerobic exercises?

    a. 90 minutes
    b. 110 minutes
    c. 150 minutes
    d. 200 minutes

42. If, when attempting to assist a patient to ambulate, the patient is very unsteady on the feet, what should the nurse do?

    a. Apply a gait belt
    b. Postpone walking
    c. Use a walker
    d. Ask another person to help

43. When using a cane to support weight while standing, about how far from the body should the tip be positioned?

    a. 4 inches in front of and to the side of the foot
    b. 6 inches in front of and to the side of the foot
    c. 6 inches in front of and 2 inches to the side of the foot
    d. 8 inches in front of and 4 inches to the side of the foot

44. If a patient has been fitted properly for crutches, how far below the axilla should the shoulder rest be?

    a. 0.5-1.0 inch
    b. 1-2 inches
    c. 3-4 inches
    d. 4-5 inches

45. Older adults need at least how many hours of sleep each day?

    a. 4 hours
    b. 6 hours
    c. 7 hours
    d. 10 hours

46. If a patient complains of chronic constipation, which dietary modification is likely most indicated?

    a. Increased fats
    b. Increased carbohydrates
    c. Increased dairy products
    d. Increased fiber

47. How many calories are in a gram of protein?

    a. 10
    b. 8
    c. 6
    d. 4

48. Tarry stools may be an indication of which of the following?

- a. Bleeding in the upper GI tract
- b. Bleeding in the lower GI tract
- c. Obstruction of bile
- d. Intestinal infection

49. If a patient with arthritis and limited mobility is sometimes incontinent of urine when the patient is unable to get up and go to the bathroom in time, what type of urinary incontinence is the patient likely exhibiting?

- a. Urge
- b. Overflow
- c. Functional
- d. Stress

50. If a patient with Alzheimer's disease tends to get agitated in the evening and at night and gets out of bed and empties her drawers and closet, what is this referred to?

- a. Delirium
- b. Sundowners syndrome
- c. Wandering
- d. Stress syndrome

51. In the first year of life, how much does the infant's weight usually increase?

- a. Double
- b. Triple
- c. Quadruple
- d. Quintuple (5 times)

52. Which of the following is an example of cultural awareness?

- a. Self-examination of personal prejudices/biases
- b. Obtaining information about diverse cultural groups
- c. Motivation to understand other cultures
- d. Assessing cultural needs as part of care

53. If using a blood pressure cuff to manually assess systolic blood pressure by palpating the brachial artery, how high should the blood pressure cuff be inflated?

- a. ≥200 mm Hg
- b. 10 mm Hg above where pulse can no longer be palpated
- c. 30 mm Hg above where pulse can no longer be palpated
- d. 50 mm Hg above where pulse can no longer be palpated

54. What dietary restriction should be anticipated of patients who are Muslims?

- a. No dietary restriction
- b. Avoidance of all meat
- c. Avoidance of beef
- d. Avoidance of pork

55. How would a patient who is biologically female but identifies and lives as a male with a female partner be classified?

    a. Transgender heterosexual
    b. Transgender homosexual
    c. Homosexual
    d. Transgender lesbian

56. If the nurse walks into the room of a long-term patient (who is mentally alert) and her visiting husband and finds them having sex, what is the most appropriate response?

    a. Leave immediately and post a "Do not enter" sign on the door
    b. Insist that the husband leave immediately
    c. Call the physician and ask for directions
    d. Admonish them for completely unacceptable behavior

57. What is the average age at about which a woman experiences menopause?

    a. 45
    b. 50
    c. 55
    d. 60

58. If a patient expected to have recovered from an injury in a month and feels like a failure because that didn't happen, which of the following is the best response?

    a. Reassure the patient that recovery will eventually occur
    b. Advise the patient to focus on the positives
    c. Help the patient establish realistic short-term goals
    d. Tell the patient that the recovery goal was unrealistic

59. If a teenager was seriously injured when joyriding recklessly with friends, what was likely the teenager's motivation to participate?

    a. Lack of intelligence
    b. Self-destructive impulses
    c. Lack of respect for authority
    d. Desire to belong

60. If a patient who identified as a lapsed Christian is nearing death but still alert, how should the nurse address spirituality?

    a. Wait for the patient to discuss the matter
    b. Assume the patient does not want to see a priest/pastor
    c. Ask the patient if he/she wants to see a priest/pastor
    d. Ask family members if the patient would like to see a priest/pastor

61. Which of the following is important when caring for a patient who suffered a brain injury and is nonresponsive?

    a. Talk to the patient while providing care
    b. Avoid talking to the patient while providing care
    c. Finish the care as quickly as possible
    d. Limit care to only that essential

62. If a parent of a child nearing death tells the nurse that the child is getting much better and the parent expects to take the child home soon, which stage of grief (Kübler-Ross) is the parent likely exhibiting?

a. Anger
b. Denial
c. Bargaining
d. Acceptance

63. According to Maslow's Hierarchy of Needs, which of the following is a characteristic of self-actualization?

a. Realistic/Self-confident
b. Dependent on others
c. Tends to be self-centered
d. Unsure about what is right and wrong

64. Who is responsible for ensuring that information about patients is secure?

a. Administration
b. Supervisory staff
c. Information technologists
d. All staff members

65. If a patient focuses energy on his family and refuses to think about his illness, which of the following defense mechanisms is the patient utilizing?

a. Repression
b. Sublimation
c. Suppression
d. Denial

66. If a patient with bulimia repeatedly makes herself vomit, this increases the risk of developing which acid-base disorder?

a. Respiratory acidosis
b. Respiratory alkalosis
c. Metabolic acidosis
d. Metabolic alkalosis

67. What is the most common risk factor for diabetic peripheral neuropathy?

a. Alcoholism
b. Long-term elevated glucose level
c. Lack of exercise
d. Overweight

68. Which of the following is the most appropriate documentation about a patient who is clearly upset?

a. "Patient angry and upset."
b. "Patient uncooperative and refusing food."
c. "Patient threw food and yelled curse words at staff members."
d. "Patient in need of emotional support."

69. If a Native American patient repeatedly avoids making eye contact with the nurse, what does this likely indicate?

   a. Fear
   b. Lying
   c. Respect
   d. Dislike

70. Which of the following is the first of the six rights of medication administration?

   a. Right route
   b. Right dose
   c. Right medication
   d. Right patient

71. If a medication order states, "Allopurinol 50 mg BID PO qd," how should the medication be administered?

   a. Orally, two times daily
   b. Rectally three times daily
   c. Orally, every two hours
   d. Rectally two time daily

72. If the nurse ensures that a patient has given informed consent for a procedure, this supports which of the following ethical principles?

   a. Justice
   b. Autonomy
   c. Beneficence
   d. Veracity

73. Which breathing pattern is characterized by rapid deep inspirations and may lead to hypocarbia/hypocapnia (decreased level of carbon dioxide)?

   a. Hyperpnea
   b. Tachypnea
   c. Hypoventilation
   d. Hyperventilation

74. Which of the following infectious diseases is associated with fever, shortness of breath, cough, and loss of smell and/or taste?

   a. Covid-19
   b. SARS
   c. Influenza
   d. Bronchitis

75. If a patient's blood pressure is 136/88, how is the BP categorized?

   a. Normal
   b. Elevated
   c. Stage 1 hypertensive
   d. Stage 2 hypertensive

76. When taking a patient's blood pressure, which of the following may result in a false high reading?

    a. Arm above level of the heart

    b. Arm below level of the heart

    c. Cuff too wide for size of the arm

    d. Inflation level inadequate

77. If an older patient reports avoiding showering at home because of fear of falls, what is the most appropriate advice?

    a. Take sponge baths

    b. Take a tub bath

    c. Install safety bars and shower chair

    d. Arrange for someone to assist

78. What symptoms are typical of Cushing's triad with increasing intracranial pressure?

    a. Bradycardia, Cheyne-Stokes respirations, systolic hypertension with increasing pulse pressure

    b. Tachycardia, hyperventilation, systolic hypotension with decreasing pulse pressure

    c. Tachycardia, Cheyne-Stokes respirations, systolic hypotension with decreasing pulse pressure

    d. Bradycardia, hypoventilation, systolic hypertension with decreasing pulse pressure

79. The onset of menses in girls is usually at what age?

    a. 10 and a half

    b. 12 and a half

    c. 14

    d. 15

80. If a patient develops diabetes insipidus after a craniotomy, what electrolyte imbalance should be anticipated?

    a. Hypercalcemia

    b. Hypocalcemia

    c. Hyponatremia

    d. Hypernatremia

81. For diabetes mellitus type 2, which of the following is usually the initial drug of choice?

    a. Metformin

    b. Sulfonylureas

    c. Meglitinides

    d. thiazolidinediones

82. If a patient with diabetes mellitus type 1 develops cold clammy skin, headache, tachycardia, tremors, and dizziness, what is the likely cause?

    a. Hyperglycemia

    b. Hypoglycemia

    c. Infection

    d. Diabetic ketoacidosis

83. If a patient has chronic elevated uric acid levels and recurrent gout attacks, what dietary modification is indicated?
   a. Decreased sugar intake
   b. Decreased fat intake
   c. Decreased fluid intake
   d. Decreased purine intake

84. In order to help prevent dumping syndrome after a gastrectomy, how should fluids be taken?
   a. With meals
   b. 15-20 minutes before or after meals
   c. 30-45 minutes before or after meals
   d. 60-90 minutes before or after meals

85. Which of the following patients would have priority for care?
   a. A patient with heart failure complaining of increasing dyspnea
   b. A patient who needs a dressing change after a nephrectomy
   c. A patient who is ready for discharge after a bowel resection
   d. A patient complaining of nausea

86. Which of the following is an indication of patient-centered care?
   a. Having only one patient to care for
   b. Developing a plan of care for the patient
   c. Informing the patient about decisions of care
   d. Involving the patient in decisions about care

87. What is the normal ratio of hematocrit to hemoglobin?
   a. 2:1
   b. 3:1
   c. 4:1
   d. 5:1

88. When should discharge planning for a stroke patient begin?
   a. When patient stabilizes
   b. When directed by the physician
   c. Immediately before discharge
   d. On admission

89. When educating a new mother about infant care, what should the nurse tell the patient about the infant's crying?
   a. Crying is a form of exercise
   b. The reason for crying is usually unclear
   c. If the mother ignores the crying, the infant will cry less
   d. Crying is an expression of need

90. What is the nurse's primary responsibility after delegating tasks to unlicensed assistive personnel?

    a. Assess completion of tasks and outcomes
    b. Document care provided
    c. Ask UAP if the care was provided as delegated
    d. Ask the patient if the care was adequate

91. Which of the following is a hypertonic IV solution?

    a. 0.45% NaCl
    b. Lactated Ringers
    c. D10W
    d. 0.9% NaCl (NS)

92. Why is normal saline IV infusions contraindicated for patients with heart failure?

    a. It may cause hemolysis of red blood cells
    b. It may increase the risk of dehydration
    c. It may increase the risk of hyperglycemia
    d. It may increase the risk of fluid volume overload

93. Which of the following foods should be avoided by a patient who must limit potassium intake because of kidney failure?

    a. Lettuce
    b. Bananas
    c. Asparagus
    d. Rice

94. Following thyroidectomy, which symptoms indicate that the patient has developed hypocalcemia?

    a. Numbness and tingling in fingers and toes
    b. Nausea and vomiting
    c. Headache and dizziness
    d. Generalized weakness

95. Which of the following can increase insensible water loss?

    a. Mechanical ventilation
    b. Vomiting
    c. Temperature 38.6 °C/101.5 °F
    d. Increased urinary output

96. If a patient has severe COPD, the patient is especially at risk for which acid-base disorder?

    a. Respiratory acidosis
    b. Respiratory alkalosis
    c. Metabolic acidosis
    d. Metabolic alkalosis

97. **Which of the following contains monosaturated fats?**
    a. Corn oil
    b. Beef
    c. Hard yellow cheese
    d. Avocados

98. **Before which of the following laboratory tests should the patient be advised to avoid engaging in strenuous exercise or eating meat?**
    a. BUN
    b. CBC
    c. Serum creatinine
    d. Bilirubin

99. **Which of the following nutrients are especially important to promote wound healing?**
    a. Fats and protein
    b. Protein and vitamin C
    c. Fats and vitamin C
    d. Carbohydrates and vitamin D

100. **What is the maximum volume of a drug that should generally be injected intramuscularly for an adult?**
    a. 2 mL
    b. 3 mL
    c. 4 mL
    d. 5 mL

101. **When performing CPR, what compression to breath ratio should be utilized by healthcare providers?**
    a. 4:1
    b. 15:2
    c. 30:2
    d. 60:4

102. **What is the correct Heimlich procedure for an adult who is choking and unable to speak or breathe?**
    a. Five abdominal thrusts, repeat as needed
    b. Five back blows, repeat as needed
    c. Five abdominal thrusts, five back blows, repeat as needed
    d. Five back blows, five abdominal thrusts, repeat as needed

103. **Which of the following is the best exercise for patients postoperatively to improve venous return in the legs and prevent DVT?**
    a. Move the feet in circles and forward (toward the head) and back
    b. Press the knees firmly against the mattress
    c. Do leg lifts bilaterally
    d. Do bicycling movements with legs elevated

104. If a large abdominal wound is separating (dehiscing), what action should the nurse take in addition to notifying other staff and the physician?

a. Place patient flat in bed and cover wound with dry sterile dressing
b. Place patient in upright position, knees flexed, and cover wound with sterile NS dressing
c. Place patient in semi-Fowler's position, knees flexed, and cover wound with sterile NS dressing
d. Place the patient in Trendelenburg position, knees flexed, and cover wound with sterile NS dressing

105. When assessing the lungs, where is the best place to auscultate bronchovesicular sounds?

a. Over trachea
b. Between the scapula
c. Over lung bases
d. Below clavicles

106. When using a bladder scanner to assess post-void residual urine, what is considered a normal volume?

a. <10 mL
b. <30 mL
c. <50 mL
d. <80 mL

107. In the first few weeks after creation of a colostomy, how often should the stoma be measured?

a. When the size appears to change
b. Daily
c. Weekly
d. With every pouch change

108. If a patient has an advance directive that indicates the request for DNR, but the patient goes into cardiac arrest in the recovery room and the anesthesiologist begins resuscitation, what is the most appropriate response?

a. Advise the anesthesiologist of the advance directive and DNR request
b. Refuse to assist with resuscitation efforts
c. Ask a supervisor for guidance regarding resuscitation
d. Assist with resuscitation efforts without comment

109. When checking the abdominal dressing of a patient in the recovery room after a bowel resection, if the nurse sees a 2 cm area of bright red blood on the dressing, what is the most appropriate action?

a. Immediately notify the physician
b. Draw about the drainage and write date and time
c. Remove the dressing and assess the wound
d. Check the wound every 10 minutes

110. Which of the following dressing types is most appropriate for a large pressure ulcer on the coccyx with copious drainage?

    a. Hydrocolloid
    b. Hydrogel
    c. Gauze
    d. Alginate

111. If using a 35 mL syringe for high-pressure irrigation of a wound, what size needle or angiocath should be attached?

    a. 16
    b. 19
    c. 22
    d. 24

112. If a patient is to have a chest tube removed, what type of dressing should the nurse prepare?

    a. Occlusive dressing
    b. Dry gauze dressing
    c. Transparent film dressing
    d. Absorbant pads

113. After emptying a Jackson-Pratt drainage device, how does the nurse re-establish suction?

    a. Connect to wall suction
    b. Close the drainage port
    c. Compress the bulb and then close the drainage port
    d. Close the drainage port and then compress the bulb

114. If a wound is deep and some of the packing is missing when the nurse removed the packing from the wound with a dressing change, what should the nurse do?

    a. Notify the physician that some gauze is inside the wound
    b. Probe the wound with cotton swabs to dislodge the gauze
    c. Use a Kelly clamp to probe the wound and grasp the gauze
    d. Flush the wound with copious amounts of NS to loosen the gauze

115. If, when attempting to do an NG tube feeding, the nurse notes that the NG tube extends 6 inches less than when inserted and secured, what is the most appropriate response?

    a. Carry out the tube feeding
    b. Hold the tube feeding and notify the physician
    c. Advance the NG tube 6 inches
    d. Remove the NG tube

116. If applying a dry heat device, such as a water-flow pad, to the skin, what is an appropriate temperature for most patients?

    a. 40 °C/104 °F
    b. 39 °C/ 102.2 °F
    c. 38 °C/ 100.4 °F
    d. 37 °C/ 98.6 °F

117. If a parent tells the nurse that the patient, a 3-year-old child, is willful and uncooperative and sometimes throws temper tantrums, what should the nurse advise the parent?

    a. The child needs more consistent discipline
    b. The child may need to be assessed by a psychologist
    c. This is immature behavior for a 3-year-old
    d. This is normal behavior for a 3-year-old

118. If a patient sitting in a chair begins to experience a generalized seizure, what is the most appropriate response?

    a. Hold patient in the chair until the seizure subsides
    b. Ease patient onto the floor and place in supine position
    c. Ease patient onto the floor, place in sidelying position, and support head
    d. Ease patient onto the floor into sitting position

119. If a child is diagnosed with intussusception, what type of stool is the child likely to pass?

    a. Currant jelly-like stool
    b. Clay colored stool
    c. Liquid stool
    d. Normal stool

120. A patient with juvenile rheumatoid arthritis taking aspirin should be aware of what classic signs of aspirin toxicity?

    a. Tinnitus, hyperventilation, and GI upset
    b. Tinnitus, bruising, and hematuria
    c. Abdominal pain, diarrhea, and hematuria
    d. Hyperventilation, agitation, and tinnitus

121. A patient with bacterial meningitis is especially at risk for which of the following?

    a. Kidney disease
    b. Neurological impairment
    c. Liver failure
    d. Blindness

122. Which of the following is a characteristic of rheumatoid arthritis?

    a. Asymmetrical joint involvement
    b. Negative ACPA (Anticitrullinated protein antibody)
    c. Decreased ESR (erythrocyte sedimentation rate)
    d. Stiffness in the morning upon arising and lasting greater than one hour

123. If a patient is diagnosed with tuberculosis, what type of precautions are indicated?

    a. Standard only
    b. Droplet
    c. Airborne
    d. Contact

124. How does sepsis increase the risk of acute renal failure?

a. By increasing the risk of glomerulonephritis
b. By causing an autoimmune response in the kidney
c. By causing clots to form in the kidney
d. By causing hypoperfusion of the kidney

125. Which type of anemia is a common complication of pregnancy?

a. Aplastic anemia
b. Iron-deficiency anemia
c. Sickle cell anemia
d. Vitamin deficiency anemia

126. Standard treatment for obstructive sleep apnea generally includes which of the following?

a. Pharmacologic treatment
b. Supplemental oxygen
c. CPAP
d. Surgical repair

127. Which of the following is a precancerous skin lesion?

a. Actinic keratosis
b. Hemangioma
c. Verruca vulgaris (wart)
d. Seborrheic keratosis

128. If a young adult female patient is prescribed isotretinoin (Accutane®) for severe acne, what patient education is essential?

a. The patient must expose the skin to the sun 20 minutes daily
b. The patient must remain abstinent and avoid all sexual relations
c. The patient must avoid all forms of dairy products
d. The patient must use 2 forms of birth control

129. How long does it usually take a synthetic (fiberglass) cast to dry?

a. 20-30 minutes
b. 2-3 hours
c. 8-12 hours
d. 24-48 hours

130. If, after a short arm plaster cast is applied to the forearm, the patient's fingers feel cool and look pale, what does this likely indicate?

a. Normal finding
b. Hypothermia
c. Impaired circulation
d. Infection

131. If, following injury to a leg, the patient's lower leg becomes very edematous, shiny, and taut with extensive bruising, severe pain, and numbness, what do these signs and symptoms indicate?

    a.   Infection
    b.   Compartment syndrome
    c.   Allergic response
    d.   Deep vein thrombosis

132. Which of the following disorders puts the patient at especially high risk of latex allergy?

    a.   Systemic lupus erythematosus
    b.   Rheumatoid arthritis
    c.   Hashimoto's thyroiditis
    d.   Spina bifida

133. When a patient is undergoing plasmapheresis/therapeutic plasma exchange, for which of the following complications should the nurse be especially on alert?

    a.   Infection
    b.   Electrolyte imbalance
    c.   Hypovolemia
    d.   Hypervolemia

134. If a patient taking antipsychotics has developed stiff jerky movements and repeatedly sticks out his tongue and pulls at his hair, what is the most likely cause?

    a.   Tardive dyskinesia
    b.   Uncontrolled hallucinations
    c.   Allergic reaction to drugs
    d.   Traumatic brain injury

135. Which of the following are the primary symptoms of bipolar disorder?

    a.   Mania, delusions, and depression
    b.   Hallucinations, delusions, and mania
    c.   Anxiety, depression, and mania
    d.   Mania, hypomania, and depression

136. What is the first step in medication reconciliation?

    a.   Check new medication orders
    b.   List all current medications, vitamins, and OTC drugs
    c.   Review the list of patient allergies
    d.   Identify duplicate medications

137. During phase I of post-anesthesia care, how frequently should monitoring of vital signs be done during the first 60 minutes?

    a.   At least every 5 minutes
    b.   At least every 10 minutes
    c.   At least every 15 minutes
    d.   At least 20 minutes

138. Which of the following patients is most at risk for polypharmacy?
a. An older adult with multiple chronic health problems
b. An adolescent with heroin addiction
c. A pregnant woman in good health
d. A middle-aged male with benign prostatic hypertrophy

139. A patient receiving IV chemotherapy for leukemia is especially at risk for which of the following?
a. Psychosis
b. Cognitive impairment
c. Infection
d. Hypertension

140. What is the most common cause of difficulty urinating in older adult males?
a. Hyperactive bladder
b. Benign prostatic hypertrophy
c. Sexually-transmitted disease
d. Prostate cancer

141. If the nurse notes erythema migrans (circular bullseye rash) when examining a patient, the nurse should suspect which of the following disorders?
a. West Nile Virus
b. Syphilis
c. Rocky Mountain spotted fever
d. Lyme disease

142. How does West Nile virus spread to humans?
a. Mosquito bite
b. Tick bite
c. Spider bite
d. Mite bite

143. Which of the following symptoms does the nurse expect to find in a patient who suffered a stroke in the right side of the brain?
a. Impaired ability to speak, comprehend language
b. Weakness or paralysis on the left side
c. Slow, cautious performance
d. Impaired understanding of mathematics

144. Where can Crohn's disease occur in the GI tract?
a. Small intestines
b. Large intestines
c. Rectum and anus
d. Anywhere from mouth to anus

145. Which dietary modification is usually indicated for mild to moderate diverticulitis?

   a. Low fiber
   b. High fiber
   c. Clear liquid
   d. Full liquid

146. If an infant has Hirschsprung's disease, what symptom is usually the first to occur?

   a. Constipation
   b. Diarrhea
   c. Projectile vomiting
   d. Bowel obstruction

147. If a patient has a PEG tube in place for feedings, what cleansing is needed about the base of the tube?

   a. Cleanse once daily with hydrogen peroxide
   b. Cleanse twice daily with soap and water
   c. Cleanse twice daily with betadine solution
   d. Cleanse daily with isopropyl alcohol 70%

148. If a client with dementia repeatedly asks the nurse if the client's husband, who died 10 years earlier, is coming, which of the following is the most appropriate response?

   a. "Your husband died many years ago."
   b. "No, your husband won't be coming."
   c. "I can see you're missing your husband. Tell me about him."
   d. "Your husband will be here later, so just be patient."

149. If a patient complains of dizziness on standing, and the nurse notes that the patient's blood pressure drops from 138/88 to 106/72 when standing from a sitting position, what should the initial response be?

   a. Advise the patient to see a cardiologist
   b. Suggest the patient use a walker to prevent falls
   c. Review the patient's diet and nutrition
   d. Review the patient's list of medications and alcohol intake

150. If a patient requires CPR, which of the following is a non-shockable rhythm?

   a. Asystole
   b. Supraventricular tachycardia
   c. Ventricular tachycardia
   d. Ventricular fibrillation

151. An Alzheimer patient is actively resistive to basic hygiene. However, in order to meet basic standards for hygiene, how frequently should the patient be bathed?

   a. Daily
   b. Two to three times weekly
   c. Weekly
   d. Biweekly

152. At which time of day are patients with cognitive impairment usually MOST sensitive to sensory overload?

    a. Noon
    b. Early morning
    c. Late evening
    d. Afternoon

153. Which of the following is characteristic of nociceptive pain?

    a. Acute aching or throbbing pain localized to the site of injury
    b. Diffuse or cramping pain
    c. Association with chronic conditions such as diabetes or cancer
    d. Burning, stabbing, or shooting pains

154. According to the three-step World Health Organization (WHO) "analgesic ladder," a patient complaining of moderate to severe pain unresponsive to NSAIDs may require which of the following medications?

    a. Demerol
    b. Codeine
    c. Morphine
    d. Acetaminophen

155. Which type of precautions is indicated for a patient with a surgical-site infection and purulent discharge?

    a. Droplet
    b. Airborne
    c. Contact and droplet
    d. Contact

156. Which of the following injection sites is the BEST choice for intramuscular (IM) administration of 3 mL of medication for a well-developed adult female of normal weight?

    a. Ventrogluteal site
    b. Dorsogluteal site
    c. Vastus lateralis
    d. Deltoid

157. A burn patient is upset and argues loudly with the nurse, refuses wound care, and states that the treatment is too painful. Which response is an example of therapeutic communication?

    a. "You should stop arguing with the nurses"
    b. "Everyone gets upset at times"
    c. "Let's talk about this and see if we can figure out a way to make the treatment more comfortable for you"
    d. "You should be happy that the burns are healing so well"

158. According to Maslow's hierarchy of needs, which of the client's needs must be met FIRST?

   a. Protection from danger
   b. Water and food
   c. Friendship and support systems
   d. Reaching full potential

159. A bed-bound patient has a 1.5-inch foam overlay over her mattress. The nurse places her hand under the overlay and finds that the foam overlay has compressed to 0.75 inch. What does this indicate?

   a. Bottoming out
   b. Adequate support
   c. Excess wear
   d. Moisture retention

160. A patient who is a Jehovah's Witness needs a transfusion of packed red blood cells because of blood loss, but his religion prohibits blood transfusions. Which of the following is the correct action?

   a. Assume the patient will not accept a transfusion and report this to the physician
   b. Tell the patient that he may die without the transfusion
   c. Tell the patient that his health is more important than religious beliefs
   d. Provide full information and the reasons for the transfusion

161. When the nurse enters the room of a patient whose death is imminent, the daughter states, "I can't stay in the room when Dad dies! I can't stand the thought!" Which of the following is the BEST response?

   a. "You will regret it if you don't"
   b. "Your father would want you with him"
   c. "I'll stay with him, and you can come and go as you feel comfortable"
   d. "Is there someone else who can stay with him?"

162. Which of the following terms is used to describe the biological effects of drugs over time?

   a. Pharmacokinetics
   b. Pharmacodynamics
   c. Half-time
   d. Effect-site equilibrium

163. When determining the burden of proof for acts of negligence, how would risk management classify willfully providing inadequate care while disregarding the safety and security of another?

   a. Negligent conduct
   b. Gross negligence
   c. Contributory negligence
   d. Comparative negligence

164. Which of the following is a legal document that specifically designates someone to make decisions regarding medical and end-of-life care if a patient is mentally incompetent?

    a. Advance directive
    b. Do-not-resuscitate order
    c. Durable power of attorney
    d. General power of attorney

165. Which of the following is advised to promote phase delay in a patient with circadian rhythm sleep disorder?

    a. Exposure to light after the time of minimum body temperature (about 3 a.m.)
    b. Avoid bright light in the evening
    c. Walk outside in sunlight after awakening
    d. Avoid early morning light, and seek bright light in the evening

166. Which of the following examples of nonverbal communication MOST likely indicates fear or lying?

    a. Rubbing the hands together
    b. Avoiding eye contact
    c. Licking the lips
    d. Slumping in a chair

167. What is a good strategy for helping a patient overcome feelings of low self-esteem related to chronic illness and loss of autonomy?

    a. Praise the client constantly for any activities
    b. Tell the client she has no reason to feel so depressed
    c. Provide opportunities for the client to make decisions
    d. Encourage the patient to focus on positive factors

168. Which of the following communication approaches is MOST effective to facilitate communication with a patient who has global aphasia?

    a. Speak slowly and clearly, facing the patient
    b. Use letter boards
    c. Ask yes/no questions
    d. Use pictures, diagrams, and gestures

169. A 76-year-old female dresses in youthful styles, acts in a girlish manner, and states repeatedly that she hates getting older. According to Erikson's psychosocial development model, which stage is she experiencing?

    a. Identity vs. role confusion
    b. Industry vs. inferiority
    c. Ego integrity vs. despair
    d. Generativity vs. stagnation

170. A patient refuses to participate in an exercise program, stating, "I don't want to do this!" When using the SOAP format, how would this statement be classified?

    a. Subjective
    b. Objective
    c. Assessment
    d. Plan

171. Two staff nurses disagree about the best way to carry out duties, resulting in an ongoing conflict and refusal to work together. Which of the following is the FIRST step to resolving this conflict?

a. Allow both individuals to present their sides of the conflict without bias
b. Encourage them to reach a compromise
c. Tell them that they are violating professional standards of conduct
d. Make a decision about the matter

172. Which of the following sensory changes associated with aging has the MOST impact on older adults?

a. Hearing deficit
b. Vision deficit
c. Decreased taste and smell
d. Decreased sense of touch (vibration, temperature, pain)

173. During an interview with a patient, what type of patient response elicits the most important information about the patient?

a. Verbal responses
b. Nonverbal responses
c. Silence
d. Both verbal and nonverbal responses

174. How often must restraints be removed and assessed for a patient with clinical restraints in place?

a. Every hour
b. Every two hours
c. Every four hours
d. Every eight hours

175. A patient is placed in the prone position to relieve pressure on the hips and spine with the head positioned laterally. Which of the following complications may occur?

a. Injury to the peroneal nerve as well as dislocation of the hip and stress on the lower back and pelvis
b. Increased intracranial pressure and increased intraocular pressure
c. Diaphragm displaced anteriorly by abdominal viscera, resulting in decreased functional residual capacity, especially in the elderly
d. Decreased cerebral circulation and ocular damage

176. With the timed up & go (TUG) test to assess ambulation and mobility, which completion time indicates an increased risk for falls?

a. 10 seconds
b. 8 seconds
c. 14 seconds
d. 5 seconds

177. Which of the following off-loading measures is MOST effective in preventing pressure on a neuropathic ulcer?

    a. Removable cast walker
    b. Foam dressings
    c. Total contact cast
    d. Half shoes

178. Which of the following is the USUAL goal of cardiovascular conditioning?

    a. Increased heart rate of 25% of maximal heart rate for 30 minutes at least three times weekly
    b. Increased heart rate of 60-90% of maximal heart rate for 15-60 minutes at least three times weekly
    c. Increased heart rate of 200% of maximal heart rate for 15-30 minutes at least three times weekly
    d. Increased heart rate of 25-50% of maximal heart rate for 15-60 minutes at least three times weekly

179. Which of the following refers to the process by which a medication moves from ingestion into the bloodstream?

    a. Distribution
    b. Absorption
    c. Excretion
    d. Metabolism

180. Which of the following patient positions is correct for the administration of eye medications?

    a. Lying supine with the head straight
    b. Sitting or lying supine with the head tilted forward
    c. Sitting or lying supine with the head tilted backward
    d. Sitting with the head straight

181. A patient on diuretic therapy develops weakness, nasal congestion, nausea, insomnia, and an irregular pulse. Which of the following diuretics is MOST likely to result in these adverse effects?

    a. Furosemide
    b. Chlorothiazide
    c. Spironolactone
    d. Bumetanide

182. Which form of documentation combines the use of flow sheets with progress notes and a list of problems?

    a. Narrative
    b. SOAP (subjective, objective, assessment, plan)
    c. PIE (problem, intervention, evaluation)
    d. DAR (data, action, response)

183. A disoriented patient hears a siren approaching the hospital and repeatedly calls out, "Someone is screaming." Which of the following is the BEST response?

    a.   "That sound is an ambulance siren"
    b.   "That sound is not from someone screaming"
    c.   "OK, I'll go help that person"
    d.   "You are wrong"

184. When entering the room of a patient who is deaf, which of the following actions is MOST appropriate?

    a.   Advance quickly toward the patient's visual field
    b.   Engage a visual feedback alarm
    c.   Wait at the door until gaining the patient's attention
    d.   Clap, tap the feet, or wave to get the patient's attention

185. When preparing educational materials for older adults, which of the following approaches is MOST effective?

    a.   Provide concise, clearly written, age-appropriate materials with a large font size and clear illustrations
    b.   Provide a large packet of materials covering all aspects of care in simplified language with a large font size
    c.   Provide pictorial representations (drawings, pictures) with minimal text of the steps involved in care
    d.   Provide a series of videos without written materials

186. Which of the following is true regarding sexuality?

    a.   Female orgasm is related to the ability to become pregnant
    b.   Masturbation is harmful
    c.   Older adults rarely have active sexual relationships
    d.   Alcohol use may result in male impotence

187. Which of the following defense mechanisms is characterized by expressing anger at family/friends/situations rather than at the true target?

    a.   Isolation of effect
    b.   Sublimation
    c.   Projection
    d.   Displacement

188. During administration of intravenous fluids, the patient complains of a sudden pounding headache and back pain, and exhibits tachycardia, chills, and dyspnea. Which of the following is most likely the cause?

    a.   Speed shock
    b.   Embolus
    c.   Fluid overload
    d.   Phlebitis

189. A patient receiving total parenteral nutrition (TPN) develops dry, flaky skin and thrombocytopenia. Which of the following changes in the TPN formula is indicated?

　　a.　Decrease amino acids
　　b.　Increase lipid intake
　　c.　Increase amino acids
　　d.　Decrease lipid intake

190. A patient receiving furosemide and prednisone has been drinking heavily and developed diarrhea. This patient is at risk for which type of electrolyte imbalance?

　　a.　Hypokalemia
　　b.　Hyperkalemia
　　c.　Hypernatremia
　　d.　Hypercalcemia

191. When a patient is following DASH (dietary approaches to stop hypertension), total fat should comprise what percentage of the diet?

　　a.　6%
　　b.　55%
　　c.　18%
　　d.　27%

192. An adult female patient complains of small involuntary amounts of urinary leakage, usually without sensation, during the daytime, especially during physical activity such as coughing, laughing, bending, heavy lifting, exercising, or sneezing. These symptoms are characteristic of which type of urinary incontinence?

　　a.　Stress
　　b.　Overflow
　　c.　Urge
　　d.　Functional

193. An inactive patient has been taking laxatives for a long time to treat chronic bouts of constipation and fecal impaction. Which of the following treatments is MOST indicated?

　　a.　Stool softeners
　　b.　High-fiber diet
　　c.　Exercise program
　　d.　Bowel retraining

194. Which of the following is the PRIMARY goal when positioning a patient for treatment?

　　a.　Providing comfort
　　b.　Minimizing injury and/or complications
　　c.　Providing easy access for treatments
　　d.　Respecting patient preference

195. Which of the following symptoms is consistent with peripheral arterial insufficiency?

　　a.　Hyperpigmentation about ankles and anterior tibial area
　　b.　Superficial, irregular ulcers on the medial or lateral malleolus
　　c.　Pale, shiny, cool skin with loss of hair on toes and feet
　　d.　Moderate to severe peripheral edema

196. When assessing peripheral venous refill time, what time frame indicates venous occlusion?

    a.   >10 seconds
    b.   >20 seconds
    c.   >2-3 seconds
    d.   >30 seconds

197. When auscultating a patient's heart rate, the nurse notes a friction rub. Which of the following disorders does this finding indicate?

    a.   Pericarditis
    b.   Mitral valve stenosis
    c.   Aortic valve stenosis
    d.   Coronary artery disease

198. Which of the following is a pulmonary change associated with aging?

    a.   Increased laryngeal reflexes
    b.   Increased forced vital capacity
    c.   Increased pulmonary elasticity
    d.   Decreased residual volume

199. Which of the following is a risk factor for malnutrition?

    a.   Body mass index (BMI) >30
    b.   BMI <18.5
    c.   Weight loss of 5% of normal weight over the course of three months
    d.   Body weight <95% of the ideal body weight for age

200. What percentage of body weight is fluid?

    a.   40%
    b.   30%
    c.   60%
    d.   10%

Answers Key and Explanations

1. C: If a patient has been diagnosed with early osteoporosis, the lifestyle change that may be most important is smoking cessation because smoking negatively impacts bone cells and leads to decreased bone density and increase risk of fractures. Treatment includes increased calcium and adequate vitamin D intake and regular exercise. Medications may include bisphosphonates.

2. B: The first-line drug for the relief of discomfort associated with osteoarthritis is acetaminophen (Tylenol®), especially for patients who are at risk of GI bleeding. If pain is moderate to severe, then NSAIDs may be taken or acetaminophen and an NSAID combined. If the other drugs are not tolerated or are ineffective, selective COX-2 inhibitors (celecoxib) may be administered, but these drugs are associated with cardiovascular risk. Intraarticular injections (corticosteroid, hyaluronidase) may provide extended relief.

3. C: When administering a tube feeding per a PEG tube, the nurse should place the patient in Semi-Fowler's position at 45° in order to prevent aspiration. Feedings should be at room temperature because refrigerated foods/formula may cause stomach discomfort. The tubing should be flushed with 30 mL lukewarm (not hot) water before and after feedings, and feedings should be allowed to flow by gravity rather than push.

4. A: If a stroke patient has difficulty dressing himself or carrying out activities of daily living, the therapy that is most indicated is occupational therapy. The occupational therapist can assess the patient's functional abilities and help the patient to compensate for areas of weakness and can suggest assistive devices, such as grabbers and elastic shoe laces, that can make the patient's life easier.

5. D: If a patient with a spinal cord injury exhibits signs of autonomic dysreflexia, the patient should be placed in high Fowler's to decrease blood pressure. Autonomic dysreflexia is a complication of central cord lesions at or above T6. Causes include urinary infection, bladder distention, kidney stones, fecal impaction, or other stressors, such as ingrown toenail, pressure ulcers, sunburns, sexual intercourse, or tight clothing. Symptoms include hypertension with increase of 20-40 mm Hg systolic blood pressure, vasoconstriction, pallor, piloerection below lesion, severe pounding headache, nasal congestion, restlessness, and apprehension.

6. C: If a patient is hospitalized with kidney stones, the nurse should anticipate straining the urine to tell when the patient passes a kidney stone and to have a stone available for laboratory examination to determine the type of kidney stone. Kidney stones may form when substances that prevent crystallization of urine are deficient and urine is concentrated. Concentrations of calcium oxalate, calcium phosphate, and uric acid promote precipitation and formation of stones (calculi). Stones may occur from the kidney to the bladder.

7. B: The underlying cause of respiratory alkalosis is generally hyperventilation. Thus, any condition that causes hyperventilation may result in respiratory alkalosis, which occurs when carbon dioxide levels in the blood decrease below normal, resulting in the pH level of the blood increasing, causing the blood to become alkaline. Symptoms or respiratory alkalosis include dizziness, confusion, and numbness in the hands and feet.

8. A: If a patient is prescribed short-term oxygen at 3 L per minute, the oxygen delivery device that is most appropriate is a nasal cannula. The nasal cannula can be used with flow rates of 1-6 L/min for those patients needing low concentrations of oxygen. The patient is able to breathe through the

98

mouth or nose and there is little discomfort if the nasal cannula is fitted properly. Humidification is generally unnecessary if the flow rate is less than 4 L/min.

9. C: The American Diabetic Association (ADA) recommends that most patients with diabetes mellitus type 2 maintain the A1c at 7% although the ADA suggests that some patients may target the A1c at 6.5% if they can do so without the therapy causing significant adverse effects or if they are younger and have an extended life expectancy. Additionally, if patients have a history of developing severe hypoglycemia and limited life expectancy or multiple chronic health problems, the recommended A1c may be 8%.

10. D: The oxygen level that indicates hypoxemia is below 90%. Symptoms associated with hypoxemia include dyspnea, restlessness, anxiety, headache, and confusion. Hypoxemia may be associated with cardiopulmonary disease, asthma, pneumonia, sleep apnea, and medications (such as narcotics, which depress respirations). Treatment for hypoxemia is the administration of oxygen. Normal oxygen saturation levels range from 96% to 100%. Exceptions to this threshold include COPD patients who can have an acceptable oxygenation saturation at 88%.

11. C: If a patient who receives chemotherapy has severe side effects, but the medication is justified because it provides more good than it does harm, this supports the ethical principle of nonmaleficence. Healthcare providers are charged with not harming the patient, but many treatments have adverse effects that cause harm, so the good that the patient receives from the treatment must be balanced against these when determining whether a treatment is appropriate for a patient. For this reason, patients must always be advised of the pros and cons of treatments.

12. B: Increased excretion of fluids, such as urine, and electrolytes at night is a normal change associated with aging. For this reason, as people age, they tend to develop nocturia. Nephrons are lost with age (up to 40% by age 85) although the kidneys can still function fairly efficiently unless disease processes and medications impair the kidneys and increase the risk of kidney failure. The kidneys also lose some of the ability to regulate the concentration of urine, increasing the risk of dehydration.

13. A: If an adolescent patient is angry at his doctor because he dislikes his treatment but insists the doctor is angry at him, the type of defense mechanism that the patient is exhibiting is projection—attributing his own strong feelings to someone else. Patients may do this unconsciously to avoid dealing directly with their own feelings. Displacement is transferring feelings about one thing/person to something/someone less threatening. Devaluation is consistently finding fault with the self or something else. Dissociation is a condition in which the individual feels detached from people or situations.

14. A: BP screening is an example of secondary prevention. Primary prevention is aimed at preventing disease, and includes fitness programs and immunizations. Secondary prevention is aimed at identifying and treating disease and includes various types of screening, including BP screening, colonoscopies, and mammograms. Tertiary prevention is aimed at controlling disease and preventing further deterioration and includes cardiac rehabilitation, vocational rehabilitation programs, and support groups.

15. D: If an older patient states that she sleeps only 3-4 hours each night, the next question should be, "Do you nap during the daytime or evening?" Older adults need about 7 hours of sleep but this doesn't necessarily have to be consecutive although patients will likely feel more rested if it is. Many older adults nap during the day of fall asleep in their chairs in the evening while reading or watching television. To sleep better at night, they may need to keep themselves awake during those times.

16. B: Lesions associated with ulcerative colitis are typically continuous and circumferential and occur primarily in the rectum but can ascend through the colon as well. The inflammation occurs in the mucosal lining but does not extend into the deeper layers of tissue. Patients experience urgency, frequent bloody stools, and abdominal cramping. Some develop fever, night sweats, loss of weight, and chronic fatigue.

17. C: The first step in the nursing process is to assess the patient. Assessment includes gathering information from the patient of others, such as family members or patient records. The next step is to diagnose, or identify the patient's problems, and then to develop a plan of care that includes goals and projected outcomes. Once the plan is completed, the nurse must implement the plan by carrying out the nursing interventions identified within the plan. The last step is to evaluate the effectiveness of the interventions by reviewing the goals and outcomes.

18. A: If a patient has an ileostomy, the normal consistency of the stool is liquid. The stool usually has minimal odor because there are few bacteria present in the stool. If the fecal diversion is a colostomy in the ascending colon, the stool is also liquid but has a foul odor because more bacteria are present. In the transverse colon, the stool will be soft and mushy. If the colostomy is in the descending colon, the stool will be increasingly formed the lower the stoma is located.

19. B: The frequency of bowel movements varies widely with some having 2 or 3 stools daily, but as long as the individual passes normal stool at least twice a week, this is within normal limits. If, however, the stool is very hard and difficult to pass, then it's likely that the patient should pass stool more frequently and should be evaluated to determine the cause of constipation. The patient may need to increase fluids, fiber, and exercise.

20. A: If a patient is scheduled for a right-sided thoracentesis but is unable to sit up, the patient should be position sidelying on the left side to allow clear access to the right side and with the head of the bed elevated 45°. The head must be elevated so that the fluid will pool distally and drain more readily. If the patient could sit up, then the patient would be positioned sitting on the side of the bed and leaning onto the overbed table.

21. D: If a patient complains of abdominal pain, the first thing to assess is the nature of the pain by asking the patient to describe it. The nurse should also observe nonverbal clues, such as the patient's facial expression and any guarding activities, such as knees pulled up or hands over the painful area. Then, the nurse should determine any precipitating factors, such as activities that make it better or worse, and ask the patient to rate the pain with an appropriate scale, such as the 1 to 10 scale.

22. C: Diarrhea and vomiting increase the risk of hypokalemia because potassium is lost though both. Some diuretics, such as furosemide, also result in loss of potassium. Signs of hypokalemia include muscle weakness, usually beginning in the quadriceps in the front of the thigh. Weakness may extend to the muscles of respiration, resulting in dyspnea, and to the cardiac muscle, resulting in cardiac dysrhythmias, which can be life threatening. Hypokalemia is characterized by potassium level of less than 3.5 mEq/L.

23. D: If a patient leaks urine when she coughs (stress incontinence) and when she feels the urge to urinate (urge incontinence), this indicates mixed incontinence. Stress incontinence results from weakened pelvic floor muscles and sphincter control while urge incontinence results from involuntary bladder muscle contractions. It is not uncommon for female patients to experience mixed incontinence. Functional incontinence occurs when physiology is normal but something interferes with urination, such as no ready access to toileting.

24. A: The first sign of urinary infection in an older adult, especially those with Alzheimer's disease, is often sudden onset of increased confusion. Older adults often do not exhibit the usual signs, such as frequency and burning on urination. In addition to confusion and agitation, patients may develop urinary retention and urinary incontinence with infection. Those especially at risk for developing urinary tract infections include postmenopausal women and those with compromised immune systems from chronic disease.

25. B: If an older patient exhibits sudden change in consciousness, including fluctuating confusion, hallucinations, and disorientation, the nurse should suspect delirium. Delirium occurs in up to 40% of older hospitalized patients and about 80% of terminally ill patients. Delirium may result from drugs, infections, hypoxia, trauma, surgery, alcoholism, malnutrition, fluid imbalance, and untreated pain. Patients may require a sitter to ensure their safety. Medications used to reduce symptoms include trazodone, lorazepam, and haloperidol.

26. D: Jehovah's Witnesses are likely to refuse blood transfusions because of religious beliefs although one should never assume that is true without asking the patient. While they often shun blood and blood products, they can receive fractionated blood cells, thus allowing hemoglobin-based blood substitutes.

Basic blood standards for Jehovah Witnesses	
Not acceptable	Whole blood: red cells, white cells, platelets, plasma
Acceptable	Fractions from red cells, white cells, platelets, and plasma

27. C: The correct procedure for replacing soiled tracheostomy ties is to leave the soiled ties in place while applying new ties and once they are secured, remove the soiled ties. It is not safe to leave the tracheostomy tube unsecured while changing the ties because the patient may move or cough forcibly and the tube may be expelled. The nurse should check to make sure that slack of the tie about the neck is equal to about one finger width so that the it secures the tube but doesn't damage the tissue.

28. A: Primary risk factors for the development of diabetes mellitus, type 2, include poor nutrition (especially a diet high in refined carbohydrates such as flour and sugar) and obesity. Those who store fat in the abdominal area (apple shape) are at greater risk than those who store fat in the hips and thighs (pear shape). Diabetes mellitus type 2 can occur at any age but is most common after age 45. Diabetes mellitus type 2 is the most common form of diabetes (up to 95% of cases).

29. B: If a patient dying with pancreatic cancer takes high doses of an opioid to control pain, the primary concern is that the patient will develop tolerance and the pain medication will become less effective, requiring even higher doses. Some patients develop opioid-associated hypersensitivity to pain, so increasing doses may be ineffective. To prevent tolerance, in some cases medications are rotated after a time before tolerance develops. Every effort should be made to relieve pain.

30. C: Typically, Food is typically restricted for 8 hours before arrival for the procedure or scheduled time of surgery. Clear fluids may be taken during the time food is restricted until 2 hours before arrival/scheduled time in most cases although protocols may vary from one facility to another. Clear fluids may be restricted to water. Some patients are further advised to avoid certain foods for a specified time. For example, those scheduled for a colonoscopy usually must avoid high fiber foods for about 3 days.

31. D: The finding of most concern in the postoperative period when an adult patient is admitted to the recovery area is BP 80/46 because this indicates the patient is hypotensive and at risk of going into shock. The patient should be immediately assessed for bleeding and the physician notified. Typically, the rate of administration of IV fluids will be increased to help counter the falling BP. Temperature is often a little low after surgery, so 36 °C/97 °F is normal. Pulse between 60 and 90 is within normal range, and oxygen saturation 96% and above is normal.

32. C: If, during the postoperative period for abdominal surgery, a patient develops pain and slight redness and swelling in the right calf, this most likely indicates deep vein thrombosis. Some patients are asymptomatic or have few symptoms. Because DVT poses the risk that a clot may dislodge and result in a pulmonary embolism or stroke, immediate attention is important. Treatment usually includes anticoagulants or thrombolytics and the use of compression stockings.

33. B: A nursing intervention that may help a patient reduce stress is to teach the patient to do deep breathing and relaxation exercises, such as visualization. Patients often don't realize that they are stressed or cannot clearly give the reasons for stress, which may vary widely from one patient to another. The nurse should avoid using clichés, such as "Everything will be all right," because that may not, in fact, be true.

34. A: Calcium in the nutritional element most necessary for the development and maintenance of bones and teeth. However, calcium is not effective on its own and works with phosphorus to strengthen bones and teeth. Vitamin D is also necessary as it regulates the absorption and balance of calcium and phosphorus. Calcium is found in dairy products and dark leafy vegetables, and phosphorus is found in most animal and plant foods. Vitamin D is absorbed through the skin from sun exposure and found in fortified dairy products.

35. C: If the nurse finds an older Asian patient trying to climb onto a toilet seat to get into squatting position, the best response is to provide a stool that elevates the patient's feet. Some cultures, such as Asian and Middle Eastern, have traditionally used toilets in the ground or floor and squat over the toilet, but it is not safe to squat on a toilet seat because of the risk of falling, so a stool that elevates the patient's feet is often an acceptable alternative. Patients who are used to squatting to toilet may have difficulty defecating in sitting position.

36. A: If a patient is unable to move or turn independently, the patient is especially at risk for pressure sores. The patient must be repositioned on a regularly scheduled basis, at least every 2 hours for most patients although some may need to be turned more or less frequently. Pillows should be used to cushion the patient when turned and the patient should avoid lying directly on pressure points. Areas especially at risk of pressure sores include the coccygeal area, heels, ankles, hips, and back of the head.

37. B: If the nurse finds a patient crying after the patient receives bad news, the most appropriate response is to say, "I'm so sorry you are upset." Depending on the relationship between the nurse and the patient, placing a hand on the patient's shoulder or arm may provide some comfort. While the nurse may be able to do nothing about the situation (bad news), the nurse should acknowledge the patient's feelings while avoiding trying to question the patient or provide advice.

38. D: If a patient is using a standard walker after a stroke that resulted in left-sided weakness, the patient should move the walker and the left leg ahead by 6 inches and then move the right leg forward. As the walker and left leg move forward, the strong right leg supports the patient's weight, and when the right leg moves forward, the weak left leg and both arms on the walker support the weight.

39. C: All patients should be assessed for fall risk on admission and then periodically with any change in condition. Patients who are older, have unsteady gait, or are confused are often at increased risk, but younger patients who are weak, have serious illness, or have seizure precautions are also at risk. Patients with a history of previous falls in the preceding 6 months are especially at risk. Patients who are immobilized have low risk. Some medications increase risk of falls: diuretics, hypnotics, laxatives, sedatives, psychotropics, antiseizure medications, and antihypertensives. Devices that tether patients to a bed or chair (IV's catheters) may also result in falls.

40. A: If the body is properly aligned and the body balanced while standing, the toes should point forward. Body alignment should be assess from the front, back, and side. If the body is properly aligned, then the patient's center of gravity is stable. The shoulders and hips should be level and the spine straight. An imaginary vertical line from the top of a patient's head through the patient's center of gravity is the line of gravity. The center of gravity is the point where the body's mass is equally balanced.

41. C: An adult should spend 150 minutes (such as 30 minutes 5 times a week) each week doing moderate intensity aerobic exercises, such as riding a bike, playing doubles tennis, and walking fast. If aerobic exercises are of vigorous intensity, such as jogging or running, then 75 minutes. Additionally, the adult should do muscle strengthening exercises, such as weight lifting, at least twice weekly. If a patient is unsteady, the patient should do balance exercises twice weekly. The patient should involve all major muscle groups (back, chest, abdomen, and extremities) in exercises.

42. B: If, when attempting to assist a patient to ambulate, the patient is very unsteady on the feet, the nurse should postpone walking because the patient is at risk of a fall. The patient may need to be further assessed or may require physical therapy to assist with strengthening and balance issues. A gait belt may be used if a patient is slightly unsteady at times but is not likely to prevent falls.

43. B: When using a cane to support weight while standing (the position the patient is in when adjusting the cane for proper use), the tip of the cane should be positioned about 6 inches in front of the foot and 6 inches to the side. The elbow should be slightly flexed so that it can straighten when the patient is walking to extend the cane about 12 inches in front. The cane should be held on the stronger or uninjured side of the body.

44. B: If a patient has been fitted properly for crutches, the shoulder rest should be 1-2 inches below the axilla so that it doesn't press on the nerves and cause damage. While standing (tripod position), the tips of the canes should be about 6 inches to the side and 6 inches in front of the feet to provide a wide base of support. In this position, the elbows should be flexed to about 30 degrees, which provides room for extension when walking and moving the canes forward.

45. C: Older adult need at least 7 hours (range of 7-9) of sleep each day. In some cases, if patients have nocturia or sleep apnea, they may find that they have difficulty sleeping at night. Older adults who are in good health tend to sleep better than those with health problems, and multiple factors may affect the quality of sleep. Caffeine and nicotine intake during the afternoon and evening may prevent a patient from falling asleep because of stimulant effects.

46. D: If a patient complains of chronic constipation, the dietary modification that is likely most indicated in increased fiber. Male patients over age 50 should have at least 30 g of fiber and female patients, 21 g. Fiber is also important for younger patients, but constipation tends to be more common as people age. Foods high in fiber include fruit (especially the skin), vegetables (especially dark green leafy vegetables), nuts, seeds, whole grains and bran.

47. D: One gram of protein contains 4 calories. Carbohydrates also contain 4 calories a gram, but a gram of fat contains 9 calories. This is one of the reasons that patients who are overweight are often urged to reduce the intake of fat because doing so more quickly reduces calories. If patients overeat, excess fat is stored in adipose (fat) tissue. Excess carbohydrates may be converted into lipids and also stored as fat, but more often carbohydrates trigger the release of insulin which causes carbohydrates to be used for energy and dietary fat to be stored.

48. A: Tarry (black) stools may be an indication of bleeding in the upper GI tract (such as in the stomach) while bleeding in the lower GI tract is characterized by red or frankly bloody stools. If the blood is about the stool but not incorporated into the stool, then bleeding is often from hemorrhoids. If the bile is obstructed, the stools appear clay colored or white. Intestinal infection may result in stools that range from yellow to orange to green.

49. C: If a patient with arthritis and limited mobility is sometimes incontinent of urine when the patient is unable to get up and go to the bathroom in time, the type of urinary incontinence that the patient is likely exhibiting is functional incontinence. With functional incontinence, the urinary tract and urination are functioning normally but something (impaired mobility, confusion, restraints, distance to bathroom) is preventing the patient from toileting. Identifying and remedying the cause, if possible, is the solution.

50. B: If a patient with Alzheimer's disease tends to get agitated in the evening at night and gets out of bed and empties her drawers and closet, this is referred to Sundowner's syndrome and is very common in patients with dementia. Patient tend to become increasingly confused and agitated and may exhibit wandering behavior or pace back and forth. Preventing napping during the daytime, limiting caffeine, and keeping on a night light may help to reduce symptoms.

51. B: In the first year of life, the infant's weight usually triples. Between the ages of 30 days and one year, the infant's growth and development are very rapid with weight usually doubling by 5 months. Infants grow in length about one inch a month for the first 6 months and then another 0.5 inch per month for the next 6 months. Some of the reflexes associated with infants (rooting, sucking, startle) fade within a few months.

52. A: An example of cultural awareness is self-examination of personal prejudices/biases. It's important to consider one's own assumptions about other people. Cultural knowledge includes obtaining information about diverse cultural groups to develop a better understanding. Culture desire is the motivation to understand other cultures, and cultural skills is the ability to assess cultural needs as part of patient care.

53. C: If using a blood pressure cuff to manually assess systolic blood pressure by palpating the brachial artery, the blood pressure cuff should be inflated to 30 mm Hg above where the pulse can no longer be palpated. This indirect method of BP assessment may be necessary if the BP is very weak or low and cannot be accurately auscultated, such as with severe blood loss or impaired contractility of the heart.

54. D: The dietary restriction that should be anticipated of patients who are Muslims is avoidance of pork although one should not assume this without verifying it with the patient because not everyone adheres to religious strictures. Orthodox Jews also generally do not eat pork. Hindus generally avoid beef and some avoid all meats. Many people are now vegetarian, vegan, or pescatarian, so all patients should be asked about dietary restrictions.

55. A: A patient who is biologically female but identifies and lives as a male with a female partner would be classified as transgender (because his gender of choice is different from that determined by biology) and heterosexual (because he identifies as male and is attracted to females). If the transgender male were attracted to other males, he would be classified as homosexual because his biological gender is irrelevant.

56. A: If the nurse walks into the room of a long-term patient (who is mentally alert) and her visiting husband and finds them having sex, the most appropriate response is to leave immediately and post a "Do not enter" sign on the door. While admittedly this is an awkward situation, people should have the right to sexual intimacy when possible, and facilities should try to accommodate those who wish to be intimate by establishing policies.

57. B: The average at about which a woman experiences menopause is age 50 (range 45-55). The perimenopause period during which hormones and ovulation decline and periods become irregular usually continues for one to three years before menopause. Most women have mild symptoms (hot flashes, difficulty sleeping, night sweats, weight gain) related to menopause other than cessation of menses, but some women experience more severe symptoms, including mood swings, sexual discomfort, and urinary incontinence.

58. C: If a patient expected to have recovered from an injury in a month and feels like a failure because that didn't happen, the best response is to help the patient establish realistic short-term goals. Patients often focus on the end goal rather than the process, but this can lead to frustration and impaired self-esteem. Redirecting the patient to process can provide the patient with reward and a sense of achievement when the patient reaches a goal.

59. D: If a teenager was seriously injured when joyriding recklessly with friends, the teenager's motivation to participate was likely the desire to belong. Identification with the group and acceptance are primary concerns during adolescence, and teenagers often participate in activities (smoking, drinking, having sex) that seem out of character and that are at odds with parental expectations and guidance so that they are not ridiculed by their peers. Peer pressure can sometimes be stronger than parental pressure.

60. C: If a patient who identified as a lapsed Christian is nearing death but still alert, the nurse should ask the patient if he/she wants to see a priest/pastor. Even patients who have long been non-religious sometimes find comfort in seeing a priest/pastor or other spiritual support person when they near death. If the patient wants to see a priest/pastor, then the nurse should make every effort to ensure that a priest/pastor visits before the patient dies.

61. A: It is important when caring for a patient who suffered a brain injury and is nonresponsive to talk to the patient while providing care: "I'm going to give you a tube feeding now, Mary." In some cases, patients may retain some awareness, and even this limited interaction may provide some stimulation and show respect for the person. Talking to the patient also provides a model for friends and family who may be unsure of how to approach the patient.

62. B: If a parent of a child nearing death tells the nurse that the child is getting much better and the parent expects to take the child home soon, the stage of grief (Kübler-Ross) that the parent is likely exhibiting is denial. Although there are 5 stages of grief, not all people go through all steps or go through the steps in the same order. Stages include:

- Stage 1: Denial
- Stage 2: Anger
- Stage 3: Bargaining
- Stage 4: Depression
- Stage 5: Acceptance

63. A: According to Maslow's Hierarchy of Needs, being realistic and self-confident is a characteristic of self-actualization. According to Maslow, needs are met in the following order (1) physiologic, (2) safety and security, (3) love and belonging, (4) self-esteem, and (5) self-actualization. The first 4 needs must be met before the patient is able to achieve self-actualization. Other characteristics of self-actualization include being perceptive and judging others correctly, being educated about the world (art, music, politics, philosophy), having a clear idea about what is right and wrong, and has self-respect.

64. D: All staff members are responsible for ensuring that information about patients is secure. According to HIPAA regulations, patients have a right to confidentiality and privacy; and all information, such as that found in the patient's medical record, must be secure so that only authorized personnel can access the information. Nurses must use care when documenting in the patient's electronic health record that the screen is not within sight of visitors and those who are not authorized to access the information.

65. C: If a patient focuses energy on his family and refuses to think about his illness, the defense mechanism that the patient is utilizing is suppression. Suppression is intentional (the patient is trying to occupy the mind to avoid thinking about something) while repression is unintentional (the patient is unaware that he is avoiding thinking about something). Sublimation is expressing unacceptable thoughts/behavior in a more socially acceptable way. Denial is unconsciously refusing to acknowledge something.

66. D: If a patient with bulimia repeatedly makes herself vomit, this increases the risk of developing metabolic alkalosis. Vomiting depletes the body of hydrogen ions through loss of hydrochloric acid in gastric fluids, which in turn increases levels of bicarbonate, resulting in increased pH and metabolic alkalosis. Nasogastric suctioning may also cause metabolic alkalosis. Abuse of laxatives by bulimics, on the other hand, leads to metabolic acidosis.

67. B: While all of these may be factors, long-term elevated glucose level is the most common risk factor and may be associated with both diabetes mellitus type 1 or type 2. Sensory peripheral neuropathy is the most common form. This reduces sensations so patients may be unaware of infection or injuries, which can lead to diabetic ulcers and even amputations. About 60% of amputation in the United States result from diabetes, so maintaining adequate glucose control is critical.

68. C: "Patient threw food and yelled curse words at staff members" is an appropriate documentation about a patient who is clearly upset because is it objective; that is, it is describing what was actually observed and avoids subjective judgements (angry, upset, uncooperative) about the patient. While it may be true that the patient needs emotional support, this is not an observation but rather a proposed intervention and should be included in the plan of care.

69. C: If a Native American patient repeatedly avoids making eye contact with the nurse, this likely indicates respect. While eye contact is generally valued as a sign of openness and honesty in American cultures as a whole, it may be considered rude and aggressive in other cultures. Most Asian peoples also avoid direct eye contact, especially if addressing someone who is older or of a higher social status, and African Americans, especially children, may avoid eye contact as well to show respect.

70. D: Right medication. The six rights of medication administration:

1. Right patient: Prescribed specifically for the patient and verified by two identifiers.
2. Right medication: Correct choice for patient's condition and matches the prescription.
3. Right route: Route appropriate for patient's condition and the type of medications.
4. Right dose: As prescribed and appropriate for age, weight, and condition.
5. Right time: Not expired (always check date) and administered at the time ordered, such as "stat" (immediately) or "every 5 minutes times three."
6. Right documentation: Completed immediately after administration and recorded in the correct format.

71. A: If a medication order states, "Allopurinol 50 mg BID PO qd," the medication should be administered orally two times daily. Common abbreviations:

BID = two times daily	PO = (per os) by mouth	IV = intravenous
TID = three times daily	R = rectal	qd = every day
QID = four times daily	IM = intramuscular	Stat = immediately
QOD = every other day	SC/SQ = subcutaneous	Prn = as needed

72. B: If the nurse ensures that a patient has given informed consent for a procedure, this supports the ethical principle of autonomy. Autonomy is the right of the patient to make informed decisions about medical care, including the right to refuse care. The Self-Determination Act (1991) formalized the right of the patient to make decisions about end-of-life care through advance directives, to refuse care, and to make informed consent. There are limits, however. In most states, physician-assisted suicide is illegal, even if desired by the patient.

73. D: Hyperventilation is a breathing pattern characterized by rapid deep inspirations and may lead to hypocarbia/hypocapnia (decreased level of carbon dioxide). Tachypnea is characterized by rapid (more than 20 bpm) breathing but at a regular rate. Hypoventilation occurs when the rate and depth of breathing are slow, resulting in hypercarbia/hypercapnia. Hyperpnea is the breathing pattern most often seen after strenuous exercises with rapid, deep, and labored breathing.

74. A: Covid-19 infection is associated with fever, shortness of breath, cough, and loss of smell and/or taste. Symptoms may vary and may also include muscle pain, headache, hemoptysis, chest pain, nausea, conjunctivitis, and diarrhea. Some develop blood clotting disorders and may have a stroke while some develop kidney failure. Many people are asymptomatic or have mild symptoms while others, especially older adults and those with preexisting conditions or immunocompromise, are at high risk. Death is generally associated with severe bilateral interstitial pneumonia.

75. C: If a patient's blood pressure is 136/88, it is categorized as stage 1 hypertensive. New guidelines regarding hypertension were issued by the ACC and AHA in 2017. Stages:

Normal	<120	<80
Elevated	120-129	<80
Stage 1 hypertension	130-139	80-89
Stage 2 hypertension	≥140	≥90
Hypertensive crisis	>180	>120

76. B: When taking a patient's blood pressure if the arm is below the level of the heart, this may result in a false high reading. Other factors that may cause a false high reading include an unsupported arm, a cuff that is too narrow for the size of the arm and a cuff that is wrapped too loosely or unevenly about the arm. A false low reading may occur if a cuff is too wide for the size of the arm or the arm is above the level of the heart.

77. C: If an older patient reports avoiding showering at home because of fear of falls, the most appropriate advice is to install safety bars and a shower chair. Safety bars in bathrooms (by toilet, tub, shower) should be advised of all older adults as the bathroom is the room in which most falls occur. Patients can easily slip, especially if the floor is wet and if they are already weak; and the added heat and steam that occurs with bathing may increase the risk of dizziness.

78. A: The symptoms that are typical of Cushing's triad are bradycardia with a bounding pulse, Cheyne-Stokes (irregular) respirations, and systolic hypertension with increasing pulse pressure. Cushing's triad is a response to increasing intracranial pressure and may indicate pressure on the brain stem. Body temperature may change as well because of pressure on the hypothalamus. Cushing's triad is often a late sign of increased intracranial pressure or occurs with a sudden increase in pressure.

79. B: The onset of menses in girls is usually at about age 12 and a half, regardless of race. Onset of puberty however, ranges from 8-13 years and tends to occur most often at about 10 years in white girls and 8.9 years in African American girls. There is a trend toward puberty beginning at increasingly younger ages. Onset of puberty in boys is slightly later and occurs between 9 and 14 years.

80. D: If a patient develops diabetes insipidus after a craniotomy, the electrolyte imbalance that should be anticipated in hypernatremia. DI is characterized by hypotonic polyuria because of excess fluid in the urine that results from decreased production of antidiuretic hormone. Urinary output is often more than 3 liters per day and urine osmolality is less than 250 mOsm. Patients experience increased thirst because of dehydration. Treatment includes increased fluids and vasopressin or desmopressin acetate.

81. A: Metformin (Glucophage®, Glumetza®) is usually the initial drug of choice for diabetes mellitus, type 2. Metformin decreases the production of glucose by the liver and helps the body to more effectively utilize insulin. As well as medication, patients are advised to maintain a healthy weight, get routine exercise, and limit carbohydrates in order to keep glucose levels within normal range.

82. B: If a patient with diabetes mellitus type 1 develops clammy skin, headache, tachycardia, tremors, and dizziness, the likely cause is hypoglycemia. This generally indicates that the patient's intake of food was inadequate for the previous dosage of insulin but may also occur if the patient increased activity (strenuous exercise) or experienced vomiting. Treatment includes administration of glucagon. If this is not available, then sugar, hard candy, or juice may be taken to increase blood glucose levels.

83. D: If a patient has chronic elevated uric acid levels and recurrent gout attacks, the dietary modification that is indicated is decreased purine intake. Purine levels are especially high in meat products and seafood, including shellfish. Meat products should be limited to no more than 4 ounces daily. Many other foods also contain purines. Vegetables that are high in purines include mushrooms, spinach, asparagus, cauliflower, and peas. Beans are also high in purines.

84. C: If order to help prevent dumping syndrome after a gastrectomy, fluids should be taken 30-45 minutes before or after meals to prevent abdominal distention since the postgastrectomy stomach volume is reduced. Additionally, patients should be advised to have about 6 small meals daily rather than 3 large meals and should reduce sugar intake and increase fat and protein.

85. A: The patient that would have priority for care is the patient with heart failure complaining of dyspnea because breathing is a critical need and the patient may require immediate attention and intervention. The next patient should be the patient complaining of nausea to determine the cause and to provide medication if indicated. The third patient is the one needing a dressing change after a nephrectomy because the dressing change may indicate problems, such as signs of infection. The patient ready for discharge has the lowest priority.

86. D: Involving the patient in decisions about care is an indication of patient-centered care, which includes:

- Ensuring care is collaborative and accessible to the patient.
- Focusing care on both the physical and emotional wellbeing of the patient.
- Considering patient and family cultural ideals, traditions, and values.
- Including patients and their family in the team providing care.
- Encouraging family members to visit and participate in care.
- Sharing all information with the patient and family.

87. B: The normal ratio of hematocrit to hemoglobin is 3:1.

Hemoglobin	Carries oxygen and is decreased in anemia and increased in polycythemia. Normal values: • 6-12 years: 11.5-15.5 g/dL • 12-18: 12-16.0 g/dL • Males >18 years: 14.0-17.46 g/dL • Females >18 years: 12.0-16.0 g/dL
Hematocrit	Indicates the proportion of RBCs in a liter of blood (usually 3:1). Normal values: • 6-12 years: 35-45% • 12-18 years: 36-49% • Males >18 years: 45-52% • Females >18 years: 36-48%

88. D: Discharge planning for a stroke patient should begin upon admission because the patient's diagnosis and condition determine the type of care and resources the patient will need when transitioning to another level of care, whether at home or in another facility. Healthcare providers have the opportunity to assess ongoing needs over the course of hospitalization and should have a clear picture of the patient, patient needs, and the patient's support system by the time discharge approaches.

89. D: When educating a new mother about infant care, the nurse should tell the patient that crying is an expression of need and may indicate that the infant is hungry, uncomfortable, wet, or needs comfort for some reason. While infants may learn over time that no one will comfort them if the cry and reduce crying, this is not healthy for the infant or the relationship, especially with newborns who have no other method of communication available to them.

90. A: The nurse's primary responsibility after delegating tasks to unlicensed assistive personnel is to assess completion of tasks and outcomes. The nurse remains responsible for the task even if delegating to someone else and delegation includes supervising the UAP by making observations and following up to evaluate the outcomes. The nurse should only delegate duties for which the UAP has been trained and can carry out appropriately.

91. C: D10W (10% Dextrose in water) is a hypertonic IV solution, which will cause fluids to shift from intracellular space to the intravascular and interstitial spaces

Hypotonic	Isotonic	Hypertonic
2.5% DW	5% DW	>5%DW
0.2% NaCl	0.9% NaCl (NS)	D10W, D20W,
0.33% NaCl	Lactated Ringer	D50W
0.45% NaCl	Ringer's solution	3% NaCl
		5% NaCl
		5% NaCl + DW

92. D: Normal saline IV infusions are contraindicated for patients with heart failure because NS is isotonic and may increase the risk of fluid volume overload. Signs and symptoms include increased blood pressure, respiratory basilar rales, dyspnea, bounding pulse, jugular venous distention, and increased peripheral edema. When patients are receiving isotonic fluids, the head of the bed should be elevated at least 35 degrees and the feet elevated if edematous.

93. B: Bananas should be avoided by a patient who must limit potassium intake because of kidney failure. Other fruits high in potassium include oranges, grapefruit, raisins, dried prunes, apricots, and honeydew. Vegetables that are high in potassium include cooked spinach and broccoli, both sweet and regular potatoes, peas, cucumbers, and mushrooms. Lettuce, asparagus, and rice are low in potassium.

94. A: Following thyroidectomy, the symptoms that indicate that the patient has developed hypocalcemia include numbness and tingling in the fingers and toes, tetany, cramps, dysphagia, and muscle spasms. Hypocalcemia occurs when one or more of the parathyroid glands are damaged or inadvertently removed during surgery. In most cases, the remaining parathyroid glands will take over, but if all are damaged or removed, the patient may develop hypoparathyroidism with ongoing symptoms.

95. C: Insensible water loss cannot be accurately measured because it is water lost through the skin and through breathing, so an elevated temperature (38.6 °C/101.5 °F) can increase insensible water loss. Mechanical ventilation, on the other hand, may decrease insensible water loss. On average, an adult loses approximately 400 mL of fluid through insensible water loss each day. Sensible water loss can be measured and includes urine, emesis, stool (particularly diarrhea) and blood.

96. A: If a patient has severe COPD, the patient is especially at risk for respiratory acidosis. Respiratory acidosis occurs when carbon dioxide levels build up in the body. With COPD, the exchange of carbon dioxide for oxygen is impaired, so the exchange is incomplete, allowing the levels of carbon dioxide to build up in the blood, making it more acidic. The kidneys try to compensate, but even if acidic levels decrease in the blood, they can still affect the brain, resulting in headache, confusion, changes in personality, and difficulty sleeping.

97. D: Avocados contain monosaturated fats, which is a type of unsaturated fat (liquid at room temperature). Monosaturated fat is also found in vegetable oils and nuts and helps to lower LDL and increase HDL. Another type of unsaturated fat is polyunsaturated fat, which is found in seafood and has similar health benefits to monosaturated fat. Saturated fat (solid at room temperature), which is a factor in raising levels of cholesterol, is found in meat, dairy products, and tropical oils (palm, coconut, cocoa).

98. C: Before a serum creatinine, the patient should be advised to avoid engaging in strenuous exercise or eating meat because these activities may increase the level of creatinine. Restrictions typically include avoiding exercise for about 48 hours before the test and limiting the intake of meat (especially beef) to 8 ounces in the 24 hours before the test. Serum creatinine is a kidney function test that is used to diagnose or monitor kidney disease.

99. B: Protein and vitamin C are especially important to promote wound healing. While the average person needs about 0.8 g of protein for each kilogram of weight (40-70 g), with a wound, the person requires that protein increase to 1.25-2.0 g per kilogram of weight. Dietary protein should be increased through the addition of meat, nuts, and dairy products. Vitamin C may be provided as a supplement to 1000 mg daily.

100. B: The maximum volume of a drug that should generally be injected intramuscularly for an adult is 3 mL. The volume and dosage should be verified with the physician if greater than 3 mL because the greater volume may irritate the muscle and may be less readily absorbed. The length of needle (typically about 1.5 inches) for adults may vary from 0.5-3.0 inches, depending on the size of the patient and the amount of subcutaneous fat. IM injections are administered at a 90° angle to the skin.

101. C: When performing CPR (following 5-10 seconds of assessment of pulse), the compression to breath ratio utilized by healthcare providers is 30:2 at the rate of 100-120 per minute. CPR should be interrupted as soon as an AED/defibrillator is ready; but, if the shock is unsuccessful, CPR should be resumed for 2 minutes between further attempts at defibrillation. The general public is advised to do only chest compressions at the rate of about 100-120 per minute.

102. D: The correct Heimlich procedure for an adult who is choking and unable to breathe is to lean the adult forward slightly, such as over the forearm of one arm and apply five back blows between the shoulder blades with the heel of the hand and, if the item is not dislodged, follow that with 5 abdominal thrusts, and repeat blows and abdominal thrusts as needed. Signs of choking include the inability to cough, talk or breathe and grasping at the throat.

103. A: The best exercise for patients postoperatively to improve venous return in the legs and prevent DVT is to move the feet in circles and forward (toward the head) and back. This exercise is gastrocnemius pumping and exercises the calf muscle, enhancing the return of blood. Pressing the knees against the mattress exercises the thigh muscles. Leg lifts and bicycling with the legs elevated are too strenuous for most patients postoperatively.

104. C: If a large abdominal wound is separating (dehiscence), the nurse should notify other staff and the physician and place the patient in semi-Fowler's position, knees flexed, and cover the wound with sterile NS dressing. This takes some of the pressure off of the incisional area, and the sterile NS dressing keeps the tissue moist. If the patient is nauseated, antiemetics should be administered to prevent vomiting and further stress on the incisional area.

105. B: When assessing the lungs, the best place to auscultate bronchovesicular sounds is between the scapula or lateral to the sternum at the first and second intercostal spaces. Bronchovesicular sounds are medium-pitched/blowing sounds and are equal in intensity during inspiration and expiration. Bronchovesicular sounds represent the air as it flows through large airways. Bronchial sounds are loud and high pitched and heard over the trachea. Vesicular sounds are soft and low-pitched and 3 times longer on inspiration than expiration and are best heard at periphery of lungs.

106. C: When using a bladder scan to assess post-void residual urine, a normal value is less than 50 mL. The ultrasound bladder scanner should be used to assess volume within 10 minutes of urination. If volumes are 100 mL or greater more than once, then further assessment may be needed to determine the reason. Scanning is done with the patient supine and head slightly elevated. Gel is placed 2.5-4.0 cm above the symphysis pubis and that area scanned.

107. D: In the first few weeks after creation of a colostomy, the stoma should be measured with every pouch change, which is usually every 2-3 days. The stoma is usually quite swollen initially and may change size as edema subsides and fluctuates. An accurate fit is essential to protect the stoma from pressure and the skin from fecal material. Templates are available to measure, but an irregular-shaped stoma is best measured by placing plastic wrap over it and tracing around the perimeter to make a pattern.

108. A: In most states, advance directives are not legally binding or can be overridden on the judgement of the physician, so the nurse should advise the anesthesiologist of the advance directive and DNR because the anesthesiologist may be unaware. However, the nurse should continue to assist with resuscitation efforts because the decision to stop resuscitation efforts will rest with the physician.

109. B: When checking the abdominal dressing of a patient in the recovery room after a bowel resection and the nurse sees a 2 cm area of bright red blood on the dressing, the most appropriate action is to draw about the drainage to show the amount of bleeding and write the date and time. The nurse should continue to check the wound frequently to determine if ongoing bleeding is occurring. A small amount of bleeding on the dressings after surgery is normal.

110. D: Alginates are very absorptive and appropriate for a wound with a large amount of drainage because they absorb drainage, forming a hydrophilic gel that conforms to the size and shape of the wound. Alginate dressing come in various forms (sheets, fibers) and when used as packing must be packed loosely because they swell as they absorb fluid. Alginate dressings should be covered with a secondary dressing and are usually changed daily.

111. B: If using a 35 mL syringe for high-pressure irrigation of a wound, the size needle or angiocath that should be attached is 18 or 19 gauge. Optimum pressure is between 8-12 psi:

- <4 psi is inadequate.
- >15 psi can cause trauma or force bacteria into tissue.

Low-pressure irrigation with 250 ml squeeze bottle delivers 4.5 psi while a 60 ml piston irrigation syringe delivers 4.2 psi. High-pressure irrigation (8-12 psi) utilizing a 35cc syringe with an 18-19-

gauge needle or angiocath provides good cleansing. Irrigation solution should be sterile normal saline.

112. A: If a patient is to have a chest tube removed, the nurse should prepare the sterile dressing in advance, an occlusive dressing, such as petrolatum-impregnated gauze or compression dressing, to prevent air leaks. The dressing should be applied immediately after the chest tube is removed and should be covered with wide tape or secured with elastic bandage (such as Elastoplast®) to ensure the dressing remains occlusive while the wound seals.

113. C: After emptying a Jackson-Pratt drainage device, the nurse re-establishes suction by compressing the bulb and then closing the drainage port. To empty the device:

- Cleanse drainage port with alcohol swab.
- Open port and empty drainage toward the port.
- When empty, wipe port and plug with alcohol swab.
- Compress bulb while holding it over a container to catch additional drainage.
- Immediately insert plug to close the port while maintaining compression.

114. D: If a wound is deep and some of the packing is missing when the nurse removes the packing from the wound with a dressing change, the nurse should flush the wound with copious amounts of NS to loosen the gauze that has adhered to the wound. In most cases, this will dislodge the gauze. The nurse should not probe the wound. If not able to remove the packing, the physician should be notified. It is safer to use one long piece of packing instead of smaller strips.

115. B: If, when attempting to do an NG tube feeding, the nurse notes that the NG tube extends 6 inches less than when inserted and secured, the tube may have migrated out of the stomach, increasing the risk of aspiration, so the nurse should hold the tube feeding and notify the physician. The tube may generally be safely advanced, but the position should be verified, such as by x-ray, before tube feedings are resumed.

116. A: If applying a dry heat device, such as a water-flow pad, to the skin, an appropriate temperature for most patients is 40 °C/104 °F. Other forms of dry heat include electric heating pads and heat packs. Dry heat at 40 °C/104 °F generally poses no risk of burns and can be kept in pace for 8-10 hours. Electrical heating pads intended for home use should not be used for long periods because they generally cannot be adjusted for exact temperature and are less safe.

117. D: If a parent tells the nurse that the patient, a 3-year-old child, is willful and uncooperative and sometimes throws temper tantrums, the nurse should advise the parent that this is normal behavior for a 3-year-old. A three-year-old is starting to be self-assertive, so tantrums and some aggression are normal but aggressive hurtful behavior (kicking, biting) should be easing by age 3. Ignoring the behavior is often more successful than efforts at punishing.

118. C: If a patient sitting in a chair begins to experience a generalized seizure, the most appropriate response is to ease the patient onto the floor, place in sidelying position, and support the head. The patient is at risk of injury and/or fall if left in the chair. The patient should not be restrained but should be turned to the side to reduce the risk of aspiration. The head should be supported to prevent neck and head injury. Padded tongue blades are no longer advised.

119. A: If a child is diagnosed with intussusception (one part of the bowel telescopes into another part), the type of stool that the child is likely to pass is currant jelly-like stool that contains blood and mucus. Typically, the child has severe abdominal pain and cries with knees drawn toward the

Mometrix

chest. Bowel sounds may be hypoactive or absent. The abdomen is typically distended with a palpable mass in the upper right quadrant. The child may vomit fecal emesis.

120. A: A patient with juvenile rheumatoid arthritis taking aspirin is at risk for aspirin toxicity and should be aware of the classic signs: tinnitus, hyperventilation, and GI upset (which may include nausea, vomiting, diarrhea). Patients may experience GI bleeding and have hematemesis. Initially, many patients experience only mild symptoms and may develop respiratory alkalosis, but as the toxicity increases, the hyperventilation and endogenous acids cause metabolic alkalosis, and neurological signs (confusion, seizures, hallucinations) become more pronounced.

121. B: A patient with bacterial meningitis is especially at risk for neurological impairment, which can include loss of hearing, impaired memory, learning disabilities, seizures, gait abnormalities and death. Some also develop kidney failure. Those at risk include people living in close proximity to others (such as dorm students), the immunocompromised, women who are pregnant, younger age (<5 for viral meningitis and <20 for bacterial), and the non-immunized.

122. D: A characteristic of rheumatoid arthritis is stiffness in the morning upon arising and lasting greater than one hour. Other characteristics include bilateral symmetrical involvement of 2 or more joints and subcutaneous rheumatoid nodules. Laboratory findings include elevated ACPA, RA, CRP, and ESR. Imaging shows joint destruction. RA stages include (1) slight bone thinning but no joint damage, (2) slight damage to cartilage but no joint deformities, nodules may occur, (3) muscle damage, joint deformity occur as well as nodules, (4) extensive atrophy of muscles and joints stiff and ankylosed.

123. C: If a patient is diagnosed with tuberculosis, airborne precautions are indicated because the droplets are ≤5 microns in size and can remain suspended in the air. Patients must be placed in negative pressure isolation rooms and the door kept closed. Standard precautions are used for all patients and any contact with bodily fluids. Droplet precautions are used for droplets >5 microns in size. Contact precautions are used when transmission is per direct or indirect contact.

124. D: Sepsis increases the risk of kidney failure by causing hypoperfusion, which damages the kidney. Sepsis is a prerenal cause of acute renal failure. This means that the hypoperfusion of the kidney that results occurs because of a condition outside of the kidney. Other prerenal causes of acute renal failure include myocardial infarction, heart failure, anaphylaxis, and hemorrhage. Intrarenal causes are those that directly damage glomeruli or kidney tubules and include burns, crush injuries, and kidney infections. Postrenal causes include distal obstruction that increases pressure in the tubules.

125. B: Iron-deficiency anemia is a common complication of pregnancy. With pregnancy, the plasma volume increases by about 50% but the red cell mass increases less so there is a deficit. Because the fetus takes iron from the mother, the mother needs increased intake of iron to compensate and prevent iron-deficiency anemia. Recommended daily iron supplements include:

- Hematocrit within normal range: 30 mg elemental iron daily.
- Maternal iron deficiency anemia: 60-120 mg/daily until hematocrit normalizes, at which point the dose should decrease to 30 mg daily.

126. C: Standard treatment for obstructive sleep apnea generally includes CPAP use when sleeping to prevent periods of apnea. If overweight, the patient is encouraged to lose weight. Supplementary oxygen is rarely used because, while it does increase oxygen saturation, it also prolongs periods of apnea. Pharmacological treatment is generally ineffective, and surgery is indicated if CPAP is ineffective.

127. A: Actinic keratosis (a scaly patch) is a precancerous skin lesion. Single lesions of actinic keratosis are usually removed with liquid nitrogen; and multiple, with 5-FU, imiquimod (immune modifier) or photodynamic therapy. Another common precancerous lesion is the lentigo maligna (dark pigmented irregular-shaped). Benign skin lesions include hemangioma (bright red/purple, dome-shaped papule or macule), verruca vulgaris (wart) (rough, white/skin-colored, plaques or papules), and seborrheic keratosis (soft dark brown or black demarcated lesions, common in older age).

128. D: Because isotretinoin is teratogenic and can cause abnormalities of a developing fetus, a female patient taking the drug must utilize two forms of birth control for one month before, during, and one month after administration of the drug. Patients taking the drug must pledge that they will not get pregnant during this time period and must sign a consent form. Patients taking isotretinoin must also avoid exposure to the sun because the drug causes photosensitivity.

129. A: It usually takes a synthetic (fiberglass) cast about 20-30 minutes to dry. Plaster casts, on the other hand, dry much more slowly over 24-48 hours. Because plaster casts stay damp longer, they are more easily damaged and must be moved with care. A hair dryer on a cool setting or a fan may be used to speed drying, but a warm or hot setting must be avoided because the retained heat in the cast may result in burns.

130. C: If, after a short arm plaster cast is applied to the forearm, the patient's fingers feel cool and look pale or the patients feels they are numb or tingling, this likely indicates impaired circulation and the physician should be notified. The casted extremity should be elevated if possible to help to prevent and reduce edema and the distal digits checked for circulation frequently. When elevating a damp cast, the cast should be supported under the full length by pillows.

131. B: If, following injury to a leg, the patient's lower leg becomes very edematous and taut with extensive bruising, severe pain, and numbness, these signs and symptoms indicate compartment syndrome. Compartment syndrome is characterized by the 5 Ps: pain, paresthesia, pallor, paralysis, and poikilothermia (inability to control temperature) or pulselessness. Compartment syndrome is a medical emergency and the physician must be notified immediately.

132. D: Spina bifida puts the patient at especially high risk of latex allergy. Patients are often exposed to latex from birth because of frequent need for medical care, so latex products should always be avoided with patients with spina bifida. Patients with allergies to latex should generally also avoid kiwi and bananas because of cross reactivity. Allergic reactions to latex may vary from mild itching and rhinitis to edema and erythema and even anaphylaxis.

133. C: While all of these may be of some concern, the nurse should be especially on alert for hypovolemia in a patient undergoing plasmapheresis/therapeutic plasma exchange because about 15% of the patient's blood volume is out of the body and being processed during the procedure. Plasmapheresis/therapeutic plasma exchange removes some components of the plasma and then reinfuses the remaining plasma and additional fluid (such as albumin) into the patient. The patient must be carefully monitored for hypotension and any indication of reaction, such as fever, headache, and chills.

134. A: If a patient taking antipsychotics has develop stiff jerky movements and repeatedly sticks out his tongue and pulls at his hair, this most likely indicates tardive dyskinesia. The patient is unable to control the symptoms. Symptoms are sometimes permanent, so if signs of TD are evident, the patient's drug dosage may need to be discontinued or the dosage lowered. Symptoms usually involve the face (twitching, tongue movements, blinking) or extremities (repetitive actions).

135. D: The primary symptoms of bipolar disorder are mania, hypomania, and depression. Bipolar disorder is a psychiatric affective (mood) disorder that involves swings in moods from mania to depression. The manic phase is a distinct period characterized by extremely elevated mood, energy, and unusual thought patterns, causing impairment in occupational functioning and social activity. Suicidal ideation is common in the depressive stage as well as usual symptoms of depression. Onset is typically in late adolescence or early adulthood.

136. B: Steps to medication reconciliation:

1. List all current medications, vitamins, and OTC drugs, including name, purpose, dosage, route, and dosing interval (including medications, vitamins, OTC drugs taken at home if patient is hospitalized).
2. List all newly-prescribed medications and ensure that the dosages are appropriate.
3. Compare the lists.
4. Identify and discontinue duplications and inappropriate drugs, being alert to those drugs that may interact negatively.
5. Create a new reconciled medication list that must be presented with the next transition of care.

137. C: During Phase I of post-anesthesia care, the patient should be monitored with vital signs on arrival and then at least every 15 minutes for the first 60 minutes and then every 30 minutes until transfer to another unit. Phase II is primarily for ambulatory patients who will be discharged home. Vitals signs are checked on admission and discharge. Phase III is for patients who will remain hospitalized but no bed is available. They are treated the same as hospitalized patients.

138. A: The patient that is most at risk for polypharmacy (5 or more drugs) is the older adult with multiple chronic health problems because chronic health problems are often treated with multiple medications. Older adults are two to three times more likely to suffer adverse effects from drugs, often related to polypharmacy. Issues include: taking too many drugs, taking the same drug under generic and brand names, taking drugs for one condition but contraindicated for another, and taking drugs that are not compatible.

139. C: A patient receiving IV chemotherapy for leukemia is especially at risk for infection because the leukemic process and chemotherapy depress the immune system, resulting in neutropenia, which may result in endogenous infection (skin, GI tract) and exogenous infection (from the environment). Neutropenia must be monitored by blood tests as there are no specific signs of neutropenia although, if the patient develops a fever, the patient generally requires hospitalization.

140. B: The most common cause of difficulty urinating in older adult males is benign prostatic hypertrophy, affecting about 50% of males between the ages of 50 and 60 and 90% by age 80. The enlarged prostate compresses the urethra, resulting in urinary retention and difficulty initiating urinary flow. Treatment may include watching and waiting (if symptoms are mild), medications (alpha blockers, 5-alpha reductase inhibitors), or surgery. About 1 in 9 males will develop prostate cancer during his lifetime.

141. D: If the nurse notes erythema migrans (circular bullseye rash) when examining a patient, the nurse should suspect Lyme disease, which is caused by a spirochete spread by ticks. The bullseye rash is one of the first signs and develops within 3-30 days of a bite. While some patients are asymptomatic, others develop flu-like symptoms and joint pain. More severe cases may develop cardiovascular disorders and/or neurological disorders.

142. A: West Nile Virus is carried to humans and other animals by mosquitoes, but the virus reservoir is birds. Crows were the first birds in which the virus was found, but it has spread to more than 200 varieties of wild birds and domesticated birds. Mosquitoes that feed on the birds ingest the virus and pass it on when they feed off of an animal or human. Domesticated animals can develop West Nile Virus, but horses are particularly at risk as about 40% of those infected die unless they are vaccinated. No vaccination is available for humans.

143. B: The nurse should expect to find weakness or paralysis on the left side of patient who suffered a stroke on the right side of the brain because the right side controls the left side of the body. The patient may also have left-sided neglect and spatial perceptual deficits. Performance is often rapid, and the patient may have a short attention span and act impulsively, increasing the risk of falls. Judgement is likely impaired.

144. D: Crohn's disease can occur anywhere in the GI tract from the mouth to the anus. Lesions may be in patches or continuous. The terminal ileus is the area that is most commonly affected, and about 1 in 5 patients has disease limited to the colon. Only about 5% of patients have disease in the upper GI tract or upper part of the small intestines. Symptoms vary depending on the site of lesions but often includes loose and sometimes bloody stool, abdominal pain, and loss of weight.

145. C: Diverticulitis occurs when one or more diverticula (sac-like outpouchings found in the walls of the intestines) become inflamed. Mild to moderate diverticulitis is usually treated conservatively with clear liquid diets to allow the intestines to rest and antibiotics. If symptoms are severe with fever, increasing pain and increased WBC count, patients are usually placed on NPO and provided IV fluids and antibiotics for up to 7 days.

146. A: If an infant has Hirschsprung's disease, the symptom that is usually the first to occur is constipation. Hirschsprung's disease is characterized by the lack of ganglion cells of the bowel, so peristalsis does not occur in the affected area. Hirschsprung's disease may be diagnosed within the first few days of birth if the infant does not pass meconium or may be delayed for one or two months. Hirschsprung's disease most commonly affects the rectum and sigmoid colon.

147. B: If a patient has a PEG tube in place for feedings, the cleansing needed about the base of the tube is to cleanse twice daily with soap and water, using a moistened cotton swab or cloth. All crusts and fluid should be removed from the skin and the tube, and soap rinsed from the skin to avoid irritation. After cleansing, a small gauze square with a T-shaped cut may be placed about the base of the tube.

148. C: At one time it was deemed important to always orient clients to reality, but this does not work well with dementia clients who don't have recall and can't process information well. If the nurse responds that the husband is dead, the client is likely to experience grief, and a short time later may ask the same question again, and again experience grief. The technique that is recommended is to join the person's feelings without addressing whether what the client is saying represents reality or not: "I can see you are missing your husband. Tell me about him."

149. D: If a patient complains of recent onset of dizziness on standing, and the nurse notes that the patient's blood pressure drops from 138/88 to 106/72 when standing from a sitting position, the initial response should be to review the patient's list of medications and alcohol intake. Many medications as well as alcohol can result in postural hypotension, so the physician may need to adjust medication dosages or prescribe different medications. For safety reasons, the patient should be advised to take a deep breath and change position slowly.

150. A: Asystole and pulseless electrical activity are both non-shockable rhythms, so shocking with an AED/defibrillator will not be successful. With asystole, there is no electrical activity. With PEA, the ECG shows electrical activity, but there is no pulse., Treatment for asystole and PEA includes CPR, IV access, and epinephrine. Shockable rhythms include ventricular tachycardia (VT), supraventricular tachycardia (SVT), and ventricular fibrillation (VF).

151. B: While adults don't usually need daily baths, they should bathe two to three times weekly. Grab bars, shower or tub seats, tub mats, handheld showers, and proper heating (to avoid chilling the patient) can facilitate more frequent bathing. Mild soap and bath oil may reduce the drying of skin. Patients who are fearful of tubs and showers, common with dementia, may receive a sponge bath or Comfort Bath with premoistened, warmed washcloths. Thick-handled toothbrushes or electric toothbrushes may facilitate mouth care.

152. D: Many people are more sensitive to sensory overload in the afternoon when cortisol levels are highest. Sensory overload most often affects those with cognitive impairment or those in stressful situations. Excess noise and activity can cause distress, agitation, confusion, and delirium. Sensory deprivation occurs when there is too little environmental stimulation because of reduction in sensory input because of hearing or vision deficits, inability to recognize sensory input because of cognitive impairment, or a boring environment. Sensory deprivation can contribute to confusion, disorientation, and depression.

153. A: Nociceptive pain usually correlates with the extent and type of injury: the greater the injury, the greater the pain. It may be procedural pain (related to wound manipulation and dressing changes) or surgical pain (related to the cutting of tissue). It may also be continuous or cyclic, depending upon the type of injury. This type of pain, often described as aching or throbbing, is usually localized to the area of injury and resolves over time as healing takes place, and it usually responds to analgesia.

154. B: Codeine. Systemic medications may be given orally or by injection into muscles, subcutaneous tissue, or veins to control pain. World Health Organization (WHO) pain classifications include the following:

- Step 1: Mild to moderate pain is treated with aspirin, acetaminophen, and NSAIDs.
- Step 2: Moderate to severe pain unrelieved by Step 1 medications may need opioids, such as codeine, tramadol, or Percocet.
- Step 3: Severe pain without relief from Step 1 or Step 2 medications may need stronger opioids, such as morphine, Dilaudid, or MS-Contin.

155. D: Contact precautions

- Contact: Use personal protective equipment (PPE), including gown and gloves, for all contacts with the patient or the patient's immediate environment. Maintain patient in private room or more than three feet away from other patients.
- Droplet: (Appropriate for influenza, streptococcus infection, pertusis, rhinovirus, and adenovirus and pathogens that remain viable and infectious for only short distances.) Use a mask while caring for the patient. Maintain patient in a private room or more than three feet away from other patients with a curtain separating them. Use a mask for the patient if transporting the patient from one area to another.

- Airborne: Appropriate for measles, chickenpox, tuberculosis, and severe acute respiratory syndrome (SARS) because pathogens remain viable and infectious for long distances. Place the patient in an airborne infection isolation room. Use N95 respirators (or masks) while caring for the patient.

156. A: The ventrogluteal site is the preferred IM injection site because there is little danger of injecting into fatty tissue, large nerves, or blood vessels. In a well-developed adult, up to 4 mL can be safely injected. The dorsogluteal site is the least preferred site because of its proximity to the sciatic nerve and large blood vessels and increased fat deposits. The vastus lateralis site is also good because it lacks large nerves or large blood vessels. The deltoid site is usually avoided because of the small muscle size and the proximity of the radial nerve and artery. Injections to the deltoid should be limited to 1 mL.

157. C: Collaborating with the patient to find a solution to a problem is an example of therapeutic communication. The other responses are nontherapeutic and can block effective communication. Saying "Everyone gets upset at times" devalues the patient's feelings. "You should stop arguing with the nurses" is a negative judgment that may anger the patient more and does not deal with the real issue. Saying "You should be happy the wound is healing" provides unwanted advice and ignores the patient's concerns.

158. B: Physiological needs must be met first, including food, water, sleep and shelter. Abraham Maslow stated that human behavior is motivated by needs, and that there is a hierarchy of needs that begins with basic needs and progresses to personal needs. People may not progress in one direction from one need to another, but movement may be in multiple directions in a lifelong process of working toward self-actualization (reaching one's full potential), which requires creativity and some degree of freedom. Failure to develop toward self-actualization may result in depression and feelings of failure. Protection from danger represents Maslow's second stage of needs (safety and security). Friendship and support systems represent Maslow's third stage of needs (a sense of belonging).

159. A: Support surface material should provide at least one inch of support under areas to be protected when in use to prevent "bottoming out." (Check by placing a hand palm-side up under the overlay and below the pressure point.) Static support surfaces are appropriate for patients who can change position without increasing pressure to an ulcer. Dynamic support surfaces are needed for those who need assistance to move or when static pressure devices provide less than one inch of support.

160. D: It's important to approach the patient/family with full information and reasons for the transfusion or blood components without being judgmental, allowing them to express their feelings. One should never assume that an individual would refuse blood products based on religion alone. Jehovah's Witnesses can receive fractionated blood cells, thus allowing hemoglobin-based blood substitutes. The following guidelines are provided to church members:

- Not acceptable: Whole blood: red cells, white cells, platelets, and plasma
- Acceptable: Fractions from red cells, white cells, platelets, and plasma

161. C: The nurse should remain supportive and nonjudgmental. Saying "I'll stay with him, and you can come and go as you feel comfortable" supports the daughter's stated desire while still leaving open the opportunity for her to spend time with her father during the death vigil. People react in very different ways to death, and many people have never seen a deceased person and may be very frightened. While many people find comfort in being with a dying friend or family member, this should never be imposed on anyone.

162. B: Pharmacodynamics relates to the biological effects (therapeutic or adverse) of drug administration over time. Considerations include drug transport, absorption, means of elimination, and half-life. Pharmacokinetics relates to the effect the body has on the drug, considering the route of administration, absorption, dosage, frequency of administration, distribution, and serum levels achieved over time. The half-time is the time needed to reduce plasma concentrations to 50% during elimination. Usually the equivalent of five half-times is needed to completely eliminate a drug or achieve steady-state plasma concentrations if giving doses intermittently. The effect-site equilibrium is the time between administration of a drug and the clinical effect.

163. B: Gross negligence. Negligence indicates that *proper care* has not been provided, based on established standards. *Reasonable care* uses a rationale for decision-making in relation to providing care. Types of negligence include the following:

- Negligent conduct indicates that an individual failed to provide reasonable care or to protect/assist another, based on standards and expertise.
- Gross negligence is willfully providing inadequate care while disregarding the safety and security of another.
- Contributory negligence involves the injured party contributing to his/her own harm.
- Comparative negligence attempts to determine what percentage of negligence is attributed to each individual involved.

164. C: The legal document that designates someone to make decisions regarding medical and end-of-life care if a patient is mentally incompetent is a durable power of attorney. This is a type of advance directive, which can include living wills or specific requests of the patient regarding treatment. A do-not-resuscitate order indicates that the patient does not want resuscitative treatment for terminal illnesses or conditions. A general power of attorney allows a designated person to make decisions for a person over broader areas, including financial.

165. D: Circadian rhythm sleep disorder (CRSD) is characterized by advanced phase sleep disorder (APSD), delayed phase sleep disorder (DPSD), free-running disorder, shift-work disorder, and other irregular patterns.

To promote phase delay:

- Expose to light immediately before time of minimum body temperature (about 3 am).
- Avoid early morning light and/or wear sunglasses and seek bright light in the evening.

To promote phase advance:

- Expose to light after the time of minimum body temperature (about 3 am).
- Walk outside in sunlight after awakening, and avoid bright light in the evening.
- Take a melatonin supplement in the evening.

166. B: Avoiding eye contact may indicate someone is not telling the truth or is uncomfortable, fearful, ashamed, or hiding something; however, it may also indicate respect in some cultures. People may touch themselves (lick lips, pick at skin, or scratch) if they are anxious. Tapping the feet, moving the legs, or fidgeting may indicate nervousness. Rubbing the hands together is sometimes a self-comforting measure. Slumping can indicate a lack of interest or withdrawal. Mixed messages, such as fidgeting but speaking with a calm voice, may indicate uncertainty or anxiety.

167. C: A good strategy for helping a patient overcome feelings of low self-esteem includes providing opportunities for the patient to make decisions. Other strategies include providing companionship and listening and encouraging the client to express feelings and concerns. Positive feedback and praise should be given when earned rather than praising everything that the person does. Telling the client that she has no reason to be depressed will invalidate feelings and may further lower self-esteem. Low self-esteem is especially common among older adults because they have to deal with so many losses. They may become depressed, passive, and dependent.

168. D: Aphasia is the loss of the ability to use and/or understand written and spoken language because of damage to the speech center of the brain caused by brain tumors, brain injury, or stroke. Global aphasia is characterized by difficulty understanding and producing language in speaking, reading, and writing, although patients may understand gestures. Use pictures, diagrams, and gestures to convey meaning. Picture charts are also useful. The speech pathologist should assess patients with aphasia and provide guidance in communicating with them.

169. C: Ego integrity vs. despair. Erikson's stages include the following:

- Trust vs. mistrust: Birth to 1 year. Can result in mistrust or faith and optimism.
- Autonomy vs. shame/doubt: 1–3 years. Can lead to doubt and shame or self-control and willpower.
- Initiative vs. guilt: 3–6 years. Can lead to guilt or direction and purpose.
- Industry vs. inferiority: 6–12 years. Can lead to inadequacy and inferiority or competence.
- Identity vs. role confusion: 12–18 years. Can lead to role confusion or devotion and fidelity to others.
- Intimacy vs. isolation: Young adulthood. Can lead to lack of close relationships or love/intimacy.
- Generativity vs. stagnation: Middle age. Can lead to stagnation or caring and achievements.
- Ego integrity vs. despair: Older adulthood. Can lead to despair (failure to accept changes of aging) or wisdom (acceptance).

170. A: SOAP is a problem-oriented form of charting that includes establishing goals, expected outcomes, and needs and then compiling a list of problems.

- Subjective notes usually quote what the client states directly: "I don't want to do this!"
- Objective notes record what is observed or clinical facts: "Patient sitting with arms folded, yawning frequently, and closing eyes."
- Assessment relates to evaluation of subjective and objective notes: "Patient appears tired. He has been complaining of insomnia."
- Plan is based on assessment: "Administer antidepressant in the morning rather than at bedtime and schedule a daily nap."

171. A: Steps to conflict resolution include the following:

- First, allow both sides to present their side of conflict without bias, maintaining a focus on opinions rather than individuals.
- Encourage cooperation through negotiation and compromise.
- Maintain the focus, providing guidance to keep the discussions on track and avoid arguments.
- Evaluate the need for renegotiation, a formal resolution process, or third-party intervention.

The best time for conflict resolution is when differences emerge but before open conflict and hardening of positions occur. It is beneficial to pay close attention to the people and problems involved, listen carefully, and reassure those involved that their points of view are understood.

172. B: Older adults are most impacted by deteriorating vision (presbyopia, cataracts), which prevents them from reading and navigating safely. Most people older than age 60 require glasses. People may be less sensitive to color differences (particularly blues and greens), and night vision decreases. Hearing impairment (impacted cerumen, presbycusis) may require periodic cleaning of the ears or hearing aids. Taste and smell usually remain fairly intact, although the ability to smell airborne chemicals may be less acute, and taste buds begin to atrophy at around age 60, affecting the ability to taste sweet and salt especially. The sense of touch is usually somewhat reduced in older adults.

173. D: The patient's verbal and nonverbal responses may be of equal importance. Patients may look away or become tense if they are not telling the truth or don't want to answer. Information elicited during an interview should include not only the patient's medical facts but also attitudes and concerns. Nurses should ask open-ended questions rather than yes/no questions and should ask clarifying questions. Providing a list of options and rephrasing patient's statement may encourage the patient to provide more information.

174. B: A nurse must remove the restraints and assess and document the findings at least every two hours. Behavioral restraints are used when individuals are at risk of hurting themselves or others, whereas clinical restraints ensure that the individual does not interfere with safe care. The federal government and The Joint Commission have issued strict guidelines for temporary restraints or those not part of standard care (such as postsurgical restraint):

- There must be a written policy.
- An assessment must be completed.
- An alternative method should be tried before applying a restraint.
- An order must be written.
- The least restrictive effective restraint should be used.

175. D: Prone position. Blood may pool in the extremities, and pressure on the abdomen may result in a decrease in blood pressure, preload, and cardiac output. Respiratory effort increases, and lung compliance decreases. The head may be turned laterally, or if contraindicated because of arthritis or cerebrovascular disease, maintained in neutral position. Having the head positioned sharply to one side or the other may interfere with cerebral circulation. If the head is turned laterally, then the dependent eye must be observed carefully for external compression that may cause ocular damage.

176. C: Timed up & go (TUG): The patient stands from a chair with armrests, walks three meters, turns, and sits back down. Patients requiring 14 seconds or more are at risk for falls (normal: 7-10 seconds). During assessment, the patient should be carefully observed for gait abnormalities, include unsteadiness, uneven weight distribution, abnormal position of limbs, and type of gait. Gait assessment also includes the following:

- Gait speed in five meters with slow gait (<0.6 meter/second) predictive of functional limitations.
- The performance-oriented mobility assessment (POMA) tests mobility and gait under different conditions.

177. C: Total contact casts (TCCs) encase the lower extremity in a walking cast that equalizes pressure of the plantar surface. The casts may have windows over pressure ulcers to allow observation and treatment. TCC is more successful than other off-loading measures, possibly because people restrict their activity more. Removable cast walkers allow patients to remove the casts, but studies show that people only use them 28% of the time, decreasing their effectiveness. Half-shoes may have a high walking heel with the front of the foot elevated off of the ground. Foam dressings provide cushioning only and are the least effective.

178. B: The type of cardiovascular conditioning should be tailored to the individual, with a usual goal of increased heart rate of 60-90% of maximal heart rate (220 minus person's age times 0.65) for 15-60 minutes at least three times weekly. For example:

- If there is an injury of a lower extremity, then non-weight-bearing exercises, such as swimming, weight lifting, or upper-body cycling may be indicated.
- If there is an injury to an upper extremity, then weight-bearing exercises, such as climbing stairs, running, aerobics, or use of an elliptical machine is more appropriate.
- Cardiac rehabilitation focuses on the whole body.

179. B: Absorption is the process by which a medication moves from ingestion (oral, intramuscular, intravenous, subcutaneous, sublingual, transdermal, rectal, inhaled) into the bloodstream. Distribution occurs as the medication enters the bloodstream and is carried to the tissues for action. Biotransformation or metabolism occurs as the medication begins to break down (usually in the liver), losing effectiveness. Excretion or elimination occurs after the drug is metabolized when the metabolites are excreted through the kidneys (most common), lungs, intestines, or glands (salivary, sweat, mammary).

180. C: The correct patient position for administration of eye medications (drops or ointment) is sitting or lying supine with the head slightly tilted backward. The patient should look up while the nurse gently pulls the lower lid, exposing the conjunctival sac. Drops are administered midsac with the applicator 1-2 cm above the conjunctival sac. Ointment is applied in a 1- to 2-cm even strip, starting from the inner to the outer, along the conjunctival sac.

181. C: Spironolactone (Aldactone) is a potassium-sparing synthetic steroid diuretic that increases the secretion of both water and sodium and is used to treat congestive heart failure. Potassium-sparing diuretics are weaker than thiazide or loop diuretics, but they do not cause a reduction in potassium level; however, if used alone, they may cause an increase in potassium, which can cause weakness, irregular pulse, and cardiac arrest. Typical side effects include dehydration, blurred vision, nausea, insomnia, and nasal congestion.

182. C: PIE: Problem-oriented charting combines the use of flow sheets with progress notes and a list of problems, numbered sequentially. A PIE note is made for each problem, at least one time daily. Narrative: Charting provides a chronological report of the patient's condition, treatment, and responses. SOAP: Problem-oriented form of charting includes establishing goals, expected outcomes, and needs and then compiling a numbered list of problems. DAR: Focused charting includes documentation about health problems, changes in condition, and concerns or events, focusing on *data* about the injury/illness, the *action* taken by the nurse, and the *response*, usually written in three columns (D-A-R).

183. A: Saying "That sound is an ambulance siren" helps to orient the person to reality. The nurse should comment on any distortions of reality without directly agreeing or disagreeing. For example:

- Patient: "That nurse promised I didn't have to walk again."
- Nurse: "Really? That's surprising because the doctor ordered physical therapy twice a day."

Making a false statement, such as "OK, I'll go help that person" in an attempt to play along with the disorientation in order to calm the patient is counterproductive because it reinforces the disordered thinking.

184. D: The nurse should always announce his/her presence on entering a room by waving, clapping, or foot tapping (choose whatever works best for the patient). Patients who are deaf are usually sensitive to vibrations, such as from clapping hands. If patients are deaf, sign language interpreters should be used for important communication (face the patient, not the interpreter). Assistive devices, such as writing materials or TDD phone/relay service, should be available for use. Alarms should have visual feedback (lights). The nurse should not chew gum or eat while speaking to the patient.

185. A: Written materials for older adults should be age appropriate, clearly written with a large font size, and clearly illustrated. It may be overwhelming for older adults, especially those who are weak or cognitively impaired, to receive packets of information to study, so materials should be provided when the nurse is there to review and demonstrate. Teaching in small increments is often better than attempting to teach the patient everything at one time. Videos are a useful adjunct to teaching because they reduce the time needed for one-on-one instruction (increasing cost-effectiveness).

186. D: Alcohol use may result in temporary impotence, such as may occur after an episode of heavy drinking. Long-term alcohol use may cause permanent erectile dysfunction. A number of drugs may also result in impotence and/or decreased libido: recreational drugs, antidepressants, antihistamines, antihypertensives (especially thiazides and beta-blockers), steroids, chemotherapeutic agents, and medications for Parkinson's disease. Sexuality is a normal part of a person's identity, but some misconceptions related to sexuality include the ideas that females must have orgasms to become pregnant or that masturbation is harmful. Older adults often have active sexual relationships.

187. D: Displacement

Common defense mechanisms:

- Denial: Refusing to believe. Seeking second opinions, changing doctors.
- Displacement: Redirecting feelings. Expressing anger at family/friends/situations rather than at the true target.
- Isolation of affect: Remaining dispassionate. Considering stress but not allowing oneself to feel it, acting calm.
- Projection: Identifying personal impulses in others. Seeing own failings, opinions, actions in others and not recognizing them as personal.
- Rationalization: Attempting to justify. Trying to find a rational/logical reason or cause for something.
- Regression: Reverting to previous behavior. Acting in a more immature manner.

- Repression: Forgetting. Unconsciously failing to recall traumatic incidents/feelings.
- Sublimation: Redirecting feelings/impulses. Finding a socially acceptable way to express feelings/impulses.

188. A: Speed shock occurs when intravenous (IV) fluids or IV medications are administered too quickly. Typical indications include flushing of face, pounding headache, back pain, dyspnea, chills, and tachycardia, which can lead to cardiac arrest. Intravenous push medications and IV fluids should be monitored carefully and administered slowly. Strong medications that may result in toxic effects if administered quickly should be given with pediatric infusion sets, and electronic flow control devices should be used routinely for IVs.

189. B: Increase lipid administration for essential fatty acid (EFA) deficiency.

- EFA deficiency: Dry skin, flakiness. Thrombocytopenia. Increase lipid intake with lipids at least two times weekly as well as oral fats (if possible) and topical fats.
- Hyperlipidemia: Triglyceride level increasing. Blood specimen cloudy. Decrease lipid administration or stop if triglyceride ≥400 mg/dL. Monitor triglycerides every four hours initially and then daily.
- Azotemia: Evidence of dehydration: dry mucous membranes, decreased skin turgor. Increased blood urea nitrogen (BUN) and urinary specific gravity. Decrease amino acids in parenteral nutrition formula or change to NephrAmine.

190. A: Hypokalemia: Potassium (K) levels decrease with both furosemide and steroids, such as prednisone. Additionally, other risk factors include low K intake (which often occurs with alcoholism) and K loss from vomiting, diarrhea, gastric suctioning, or diaphoresis. Potassium is the primary electrolyte in intracellular fluid with about 98% inside cells and only 2% in extracellular fluid, although this small amount is important for neuromuscular activity. Potassium influences activity of the skeletal and cardiac muscles. The K level is dependent upon adequate renal functioning because 80% is excreted through the kidneys and 20% through the bowels and sweat:

- Normal: 3.5-5.5 mEq/L.
- Hypokalemia: <3.5 mEq/L. Critical value: <2.5 mEq/L.

191. D: DASH nutrient goals (based on a 2100-calorie diet) include the following:

- Total fat: 27%; saturated fat: 6%.
- Protein: 18%; carbohydrates: 55%.
- Cholesterol: 150 mg.
- Sodium: 1500 to 2300 mg; K: 4700 mg; calcium: 1250 mg; magnesium: 500 mg; fiber: 30 g.

192. A: Stress incontinence. Other types include the following:

- Urge incontinence: Moderate to large amounts of involuntary urinary leakage caused by the sudden urge to urinate and the inability to hold the urine; it is associated with frequency and nocturia more than twice nightly and small bladder capacity.
- Overflow incontinence: Usually small leakages of urine, similar to stress incontinence, but resulting from pressure on an overdistended bladder with difficulty initiating flow and dribbling after urination because the bladder has not emptied.
- Functional incontinence: Leakage of urine because of the inability of the person to manage toileting or remove clothing for a variety of reasons.

193. D: Bowel retraining strategies include the following:

- Keeping a bowel diary for a week.
- Modifying the diet and fluid intake to assure normal stool consistency, including increased fiber and fluids, eating meals at scheduled times, and avoiding foods that increase bowel dysfunction.
- Establishing a schedule for defecation, preferably at the same time each day and about 20-30 minutes after a meal.
- Practicing Kegel exercises.
- Using a stimulus to promote defecation, such as enemas, suppositories, or laxatives in the beginning, with a goal to decrease such use. Digital stimulation or hot drinks may be used.
- Keeping a record of stool consistency and evacuation.

194. B: Patient positioning for treatments is determined by members of the medical team, such as the physician and nurses, depending upon the particular needs of the patient. The primary goal is to position the patient so that there is minimal injury/complications. Risk factors must be considered. These include age (young or old), diabetes, obesity, malnourishment, dehydration, cardiac and/or respiratory disease, musculoskeletal diseases, limited mobility, renal failure, paralysis, and duration. Of primary concern is the cardiorespiratory response to positioning because the changes in position, such as from standing to supine, can result in a decrease in heart rate, stroke volume, and output.

195. C: Peripheral arterial insufficiency is characterized by pale, shiny, cool skin with a loss of hair on the toes and feet. Pain ranges from intermittent claudication to severe, constant pain. Peripheral pulses are weak or absent. The skin color changes from pallor of the foot on elevation to rubor on dependency. Edema is minimal. Ulcers are usually painful, deep, circular, and often necrotic on toe tips, toe webs, heels, or other pressure areas. Venous insufficiency is characterized by hyperpigmentation, superficial irregular ulcers on medial or lateral malleolus, and moderate to severe peripheral edema.

196. B: Venous refill time: Venous occlusion is indicated with times >20 seconds. Begin with the patient lying supine for a few moments, and then have the patient sit with the feet dependent. Observe the veins on the dorsum of the foot, and count the seconds before normal filling. Capillary refill: Grasp the toenail bed between the thumb and index finger, and apply pressure for several seconds to cause blanching. Release the nail, and count the seconds until the nail regains normal color. Arterial occlusion is indicated with times over two to three seconds. Check both feet and more than one nail bed.

197. A: Friction rub: Harsh, grating sound heard in systole and diastole with pericarditis. Opening snap: Unusual, high-pitched sound occurring after S2 with stenosis of the mitral valve from rheumatic heart disease. Ejection click: Brief, high-pitched sound occurring immediately after S1 with stenosis of the aortic valve. Gallop rhythm: S4 occurs before S1 and occurs with ventricular hypertrophy, such as from coronary artery disease, hypertension, or aortic valve stenosis. Murmur: Sound caused by turbulent blood flow from stenotic or malfunctioning valves, congenital defects, or increased blood flow.

198. D: Typically, with age there is decreased pulmonary elasticity and decreases in residual volume, alveolar surface area with alveolar distension, and arterial oxygen tension with increased closing capacity, ventilation/perfusion mismatching, and chest wall rigidity, so the exchange of oxygen is impaired. Forced expiratory volume (FEV) and forced vital capacity (FVC) are reduced.

Overall strength is often decreased, so there is less ability to breathe deeply, and the cough reflex and ciliary action are decreased. Protective laryngeal reflexes are diminished.

199. B: Risk factors for malnutrition include the following:

- Low body mass index (BMI) of <18.5.
- Hypermetabolism resulting from various diseases, such as AIDS, and trauma, stress, or infection.
- Weight loss, especially sudden or a loss of 10% of normal weight over a three-month period.
- Low body weight of <90% of ideal body weight for age.
- Malabsorption of nutrients caused by diseases such as chronic failure of kidneys or liver.
- Food intolerances, such as lactose intolerance or celiac disease.
- Dietary restrictions, such as limiting of protein with kidney failure.
- Functional limitations, such as inability to feed oneself or a lack of dentures.

200. C: According to the 60-40-20 rule, approximately 60% of body weight is from fluid, with about 40% from intracellular fluids (ICFs), such as fluids within the cells, and 20% from extracellular fluids (ECFs), such as interstitial fluid, plasma, and transcellular fluid (digestive juices and mucus). Plasma comprises about 25% of the ECF, interstitial fluid about 75%, and transcellular fluid about 1-2 liters. The fluid compartments are separated by semipermeable membranes that allow fluid and solutes (electrolytes and other substances) to move by osmosis. Fluid also moves through diffusion, filtration, and active transport.

How to Overcome Test Anxiety

Just the thought of taking a test is enough to make most people a little nervous. A test is an important event that can have a long-term impact on your future, so it's important to take it seriously and it's natural to feel anxious about performing well. But just because anxiety is normal, that doesn't mean that it's helpful in test taking, or that you should simply accept it as part of your life. Anxiety can have a variety of effects. These effects can be mild, like making you feel slightly nervous, or severe, like blocking your ability to focus or remember even a simple detail.

If you experience test anxiety—whether severe or mild—it's important to know how to beat it. To discover this, first you need to understand what causes test anxiety.

Causes of Test Anxiety

While we often think of anxiety as an uncontrollable emotional state, it can actually be caused by simple, practical things. One of the most common causes of test anxiety is that a person does not feel adequately prepared for their test. This feeling can be the result of many different issues such as poor study habits or lack of organization, but the most common culprit is time management. Starting to study too late, failing to organize your study time to cover all of the material, or being distracted while you study will mean that you're not well prepared for the test. This may lead to cramming the night before, which will cause you to be physically and mentally exhausted for the test. Poor time management also contributes to feelings of stress, fear, and hopelessness as you realize you are not well prepared but don't know what to do about it.

Other times, test anxiety is not related to your preparation for the test but comes from unresolved fear. This may be a past failure on a test, or poor performance on tests in general. It may come from comparing yourself to others who seem to be performing better or from the stress of living up to expectations. Anxiety may be driven by fears of the future—how failure on this test would affect your educational and career goals. These fears are often completely irrational, but they can still negatively impact your test performance.

> **Review Video: 3 Reasons You Have Test Anxiety**
> Visit mometrix.com/academy and enter code: 428468

Elements of Test Anxiety

As mentioned earlier, test anxiety is considered to be an emotional state, but it has physical and mental components as well. Sometimes you may not even realize that you are suffering from test anxiety until you notice the physical symptoms. These can include trembling hands, rapid heartbeat, sweating, nausea, and tense muscles. Extreme anxiety may lead to fainting or vomiting. Obviously, any of these symptoms can have a negative impact on testing. It is important to recognize them as soon as they begin to occur so that you can address the problem before it damages your performance.

> **Review Video: 3 Ways to Tell You Have Test Anxiety**
> Visit mometrix.com/academy and enter code: 927847

The mental components of test anxiety include trouble focusing and inability to remember learned information. During a test, your mind is on high alert, which can help you recall information and stay focused for an extended period of time. However, anxiety interferes with your mind's natural processes, causing you to blank out, even on the questions you know well. The strain of testing during anxiety makes it difficult to stay focused, especially on a test that may take several hours. Extreme anxiety can take a huge mental toll, making it difficult not only to recall test information but even to understand the test questions or pull your thoughts together.

> **Review Video: How Test Anxiety Affects Memory**
> Visit mometrix.com/academy and enter code: 609003

Effects of Test Anxiety

Test anxiety is like a disease—if left untreated, it will get progressively worse. Anxiety leads to poor performance, and this reinforces the feelings of fear and failure, which in turn lead to poor performances on subsequent tests. It can grow from a mild nervousness to a crippling condition. If allowed to progress, test anxiety can have a big impact on your schooling, and consequently on your future.

Test anxiety can spread to other parts of your life. Anxiety on tests can become anxiety in any stressful situation, and blanking on a test can turn into panicking in a job situation. But fortunately, you don't have to let anxiety rule your testing and determine your grades. There are a number of relatively simple steps you can take to move past anxiety and function normally on a test and in the rest of life.

> **Review Video: How Test Anxiety Impacts Your Grades**
> Visit mometrix.com/academy and enter code: 939819

Physical Steps for Beating Test Anxiety

While test anxiety is a serious problem, the good news is that it can be overcome. It doesn't have to control your ability to think and remember information. While it may take time, you can begin taking steps today to beat anxiety.

Just as your first hint that you may be struggling with anxiety comes from the physical symptoms, the first step to treating it is also physical. Rest is crucial for having a clear, strong mind. If you are tired, it is much easier to give in to anxiety. But if you establish good sleep habits, your body and mind will be ready to perform optimally, without the strain of exhaustion. Additionally, sleeping well helps you to retain information better, so you're more likely to recall the answers when you see the test questions.

Getting good sleep means more than going to bed on time. It's important to allow your brain time to relax. Take study breaks from time to time so it doesn't get overworked, and don't study right before bed. Take time to rest your mind before trying to rest your body, or you may find it difficult to fall asleep.

> **Review Video: The Importance of Sleep for Your Brain**
> Visit mometrix.com/academy and enter code: 319338

Along with sleep, other aspects of physical health are important in preparing for a test. Good nutrition is vital for good brain function. Sugary foods and drinks may give a burst of energy but this burst is followed by a crash, both physically and emotionally. Instead, fuel your body with protein and vitamin-rich foods.

Also, drink plenty of water. Dehydration can lead to headaches and exhaustion, especially if your brain is already under stress from the rigors of the test. Particularly if your test is a long one, drink water during the breaks. And if possible, take an energy-boosting snack to eat between sections.

> **Review Video: How Diet Can Affect your Mood**
> Visit mometrix.com/academy and enter code: 624317

Along with sleep and diet, a third important part of physical health is exercise. Maintaining a steady workout schedule is helpful, but even taking 5-minute study breaks to walk can help get your blood pumping faster and clear your head. Exercise also releases endorphins, which contribute to a positive feeling and can help combat test anxiety.

When you nurture your physical health, you are also contributing to your mental health. If your body is healthy, your mind is much more likely to be healthy as well. So take time to rest, nourish your body with healthy food and water, and get moving as much as possible. Taking these physical steps will make you stronger and more able to take the mental steps necessary to overcome test anxiety.

Mental Steps for Beating Test Anxiety

Working on the mental side of test anxiety can be more challenging, but as with the physical side, there are clear steps you can take to overcome it. As mentioned earlier, test anxiety often stems from lack of preparation, so the obvious solution is to prepare for the test. Effective studying may be the most important weapon you have for beating test anxiety, but you can and should employ several other mental tools to combat fear.

First, boost your confidence by reminding yourself of past success—tests or projects that you aced. If you're putting as much effort into preparing for this test as you did for those, there's no reason you should expect to fail here. Work hard to prepare; then trust your preparation.

Second, surround yourself with encouraging people. It can be helpful to find a study group, but be sure that the people you're around will encourage a positive attitude. If you spend time with others who are anxious or cynical, this will only contribute to your own anxiety. Look for others who are motivated to study hard from a desire to succeed, not from a fear of failure.

Third, reward yourself. A test is physically and mentally tiring, even without anxiety, and it can be helpful to have something to look forward to. Plan an activity following the test, regardless of the outcome, such as going to a movie or getting ice cream.

When you are taking the test, if you find yourself beginning to feel anxious, remind yourself that you know the material. Visualize successfully completing the test. Then take a few deep, relaxing breaths and return to it. Work through the questions carefully but with confidence, knowing that you are capable of succeeding.

Developing a healthy mental approach to test taking will also aid in other areas of life. Test anxiety affects more than just the actual test—it can be damaging to your mental health and even contribute to depression. It's important to beat test anxiety before it becomes a problem for more than testing.

> **Review Video: <u>Test Anxiety and Depression</u>**
> Visit mometrix.com/academy and enter code: 904704

Study Strategy

Being prepared for the test is necessary to combat anxiety, but what does being prepared look like? You may study for hours on end and still not feel prepared. What you need is a strategy for test prep. The next few pages outline our recommended steps to help you plan out and conquer the challenge of preparation.

STEP 1: SCOPE OUT THE TEST

Learn everything you can about the format (multiple choice, essay, etc.) and what will be on the test. Gather any study materials, course outlines, or sample exams that may be available. Not only will this help you to prepare, but knowing what to expect can help to alleviate test anxiety.

STEP 2: MAP OUT THE MATERIAL

Look through the textbook or study guide and make note of how many chapters or sections it has. Then divide these over the time you have. For example, if a book has 15 chapters and you have five days to study, you need to cover three chapters each day. Even better, if you have the time, leave an extra day at the end for overall review after you have gone through the material in depth.

If time is limited, you may need to prioritize the material. Look through it and make note of which sections you think you already have a good grasp on, and which need review. While you are studying, skim quickly through the familiar sections and take more time on the challenging parts. Write out your plan so you don't get lost as you go. Having a written plan also helps you feel more in control of the study, so anxiety is less likely to arise from feeling overwhelmed at the amount to cover.

STEP 3: GATHER YOUR TOOLS

Decide what study method works best for you. Do you prefer to highlight in the book as you study and then go back over the highlighted portions? Or do you type out notes of the important information? Or is it helpful to make flashcards that you can carry with you? Assemble the pens, index cards, highlighters, post-it notes, and any other materials you may need so you won't be distracted by getting up to find things while you study.

If you're having a hard time retaining the information or organizing your notes, experiment with different methods. For example, try color-coding by subject with colored pens, highlighters, or post-it notes. If you learn better by hearing, try recording yourself reading your notes so you can listen while in the car, working out, or simply sitting at your desk. Ask a friend to quiz you from your flashcards, or try teaching someone the material to solidify it in your mind.

STEP 4: CREATE YOUR ENVIRONMENT

It's important to avoid distractions while you study. This includes both the obvious distractions like visitors and the subtle distractions like an uncomfortable chair (or a too-comfortable couch that makes you want to fall asleep). Set up the best study environment possible: good lighting and a comfortable work area. If background music helps you focus, you may want to turn it on, but otherwise keep the room quiet. If you are using a computer to take notes, be sure you don't have any other windows open, especially applications like social media, games, or anything else that could distract you. Silence your phone and turn off notifications. Be sure to keep water close by so you stay hydrated while you study (but avoid unhealthy drinks and snacks).

Also, take into account the best time of day to study. Are you freshest first thing in the morning? Try to set aside some time then to work through the material. Is your mind clearer in the afternoon or evening? Schedule your study session then. Another method is to study at the same time of day that you will take the test, so that your brain gets used to working on the material at that time and will be ready to focus at test time.

STEP 5: STUDY!

Once you have done all the study preparation, it's time to settle into the actual studying. Sit down, take a few moments to settle your mind so you can focus, and begin to follow your study plan. Don't give in to distractions or let yourself procrastinate. This is your time to prepare so you'll be ready to fearlessly approach the test. Make the most of the time and stay focused.

Of course, you don't want to burn out. If you study too long you may find that you're not retaining the information very well. Take regular study breaks. For example, taking five minutes out of every hour to walk briskly, breathing deeply and swinging your arms, can help your mind stay fresh.

As you get to the end of each chapter or section, it's a good idea to do a quick review. Remind yourself of what you learned and work on any difficult parts. When you feel that you've mastered the material, move on to the next part. At the end of your study session, briefly skim through your notes again.

But while review is helpful, cramming last minute is NOT. If at all possible, work ahead so that you won't need to fit all your study into the last day. Cramming overloads your brain with more information than it can process and retain, and your tired mind may struggle to recall even previously learned information when it is overwhelmed with last-minute study. Also, the urgent nature of cramming and the stress placed on your brain contribute to anxiety. You'll be more likely to go to the test feeling unprepared and having trouble thinking clearly.

So don't cram, and don't stay up late before the test, even just to review your notes at a leisurely pace. Your brain needs rest more than it needs to go over the information again. In fact, plan to finish your studies by noon or early afternoon the day before the test. Give your brain the rest of the day to relax or focus on other things, and get a good night's sleep. Then you will be fresh for the test and better able to recall what you've studied.

STEP 6: TAKE A PRACTICE TEST

Many courses offer sample tests, either online or in the study materials. This is an excellent resource to check whether you have mastered the material, as well as to prepare for the test format and environment.

Check the test format ahead of time: the number of questions, the type (multiple choice, free response, etc.), and the time limit. Then create a plan for working through them. For example, if you have 30 minutes to take a 60-question test, your limit is 30 seconds per question. Spend less time on the questions you know well so that you can take more time on the difficult ones.

If you have time to take several practice tests, take the first one open book, with no time limit. Work through the questions at your own pace and make sure you fully understand them. Gradually work up to taking a test under test conditions: sit at a desk with all study materials put away and set a timer. Pace yourself to make sure you finish the test with time to spare and go back to check your answers if you have time.

After each test, check your answers. On the questions you missed, be sure you understand why you missed them. Did you misread the question (tests can use tricky wording)? Did you forget the information? Or was it something you hadn't learned? Go back and study any shaky areas that the practice tests reveal.

Taking these tests not only helps with your grade, but also aids in combating test anxiety. If you're already used to the test conditions, you're less likely to worry about it, and working through tests until you're scoring well gives you a confidence boost. Go through the practice tests until you feel comfortable, and then you can go into the test knowing that you're ready for it.

Test Tips

On test day, you should be confident, knowing that you've prepared well and are ready to answer the questions. But aside from preparation, there are several test day strategies you can employ to maximize your performance.

First, as stated before, get a good night's sleep the night before the test (and for several nights before that, if possible). Go into the test with a fresh, alert mind rather than staying up late to study.

Try not to change too much about your normal routine on the day of the test. It's important to eat a nutritious breakfast, but if you normally don't eat breakfast at all, consider eating just a protein bar. If you're a coffee drinker, go ahead and have your normal coffee. Just make sure you time it so that the caffeine doesn't wear off right in the middle of your test. Avoid sugary beverages, and drink enough water to stay hydrated but not so much that you need a restroom break 10 minutes into the test. If your test isn't first thing in the morning, consider going for a walk or doing a light workout before the test to get your blood flowing.

Allow yourself enough time to get ready, and leave for the test with plenty of time to spare so you won't have the anxiety of scrambling to arrive in time. Another reason to be early is to select a good seat. It's helpful to sit away from doors and windows, which can be distracting. Find a good seat, get out your supplies, and settle your mind before the test begins.

When the test begins, start by going over the instructions carefully, even if you already know what to expect. Make sure you avoid any careless mistakes by following the directions.

Then begin working through the questions, pacing yourself as you've practiced. If you're not sure on an answer, don't spend too much time on it, and don't let it shake your confidence. Either skip it and come back later, or eliminate as many wrong answers as possible and guess among the remaining ones. Don't dwell on these questions as you continue—put them out of your mind and focus on what lies ahead.

Be sure to read all of the answer choices, even if you're sure the first one is the right answer. Sometimes you'll find a better one if you keep reading. But don't second-guess yourself if you do immediately know the answer. Your gut instinct is usually right. Don't let test anxiety rob you of the information you know.

If you have time at the end of the test (and if the test format allows), go back and review your answers. Be cautious about changing any, since your first instinct tends to be correct, but make sure you didn't misread any of the questions or accidentally mark the wrong answer choice. Look over any you skipped and make an educated guess.

At the end, leave the test feeling confident. You've done your best, so don't waste time worrying about your performance or wishing you could change anything. Instead, celebrate the successful completion of this test. And finally, use this test to learn how to deal with anxiety even better next time.

> **Review Video: 5 Tips to Beat Test Anxiety**
> Visit mometrix.com/academy and enter code: 570656

Important Qualification

Not all anxiety is created equal. If your test anxiety is causing major issues in your life beyond the classroom or testing center, or if you are experiencing troubling physical symptoms related to your anxiety, it may be a sign of a serious physiological or psychological condition. If this sounds like your situation, we strongly encourage you to seek professional help.

Thank You

We at Mometrix would like to extend our heartfelt thanks to you, our friend and patron, for allowing us to play a part in your journey. It is a privilege to serve people from all walks of life who are unified in their commitment to building the best future they can for themselves.

The preparation you devote to these important testing milestones may be the most valuable educational opportunity you have for making a real difference in your life. We encourage you to put your heart into it—that feeling of succeeding, overcoming, and yes, conquering will be well worth the hours you've invested.

We want to hear your story, your struggles and your successes, and if you see any opportunities for us to improve our materials so we can help others even more effectively in the future, please share that with us as well. **The team at Mometrix would be absolutely thrilled to hear from you!** So please, send us an email (support@mometrix.com) and let's stay in touch.

> **If you'd like some additional help, check out these other resources we offer for your exam:**
> **http://MometrixFlashcards.com/NursingACE**

136

Additional Bonus Material

Due to our efforts to try to keep this book to a manageable length, we've created a link that will give you access to all of your additional bonus material:

[**mometrix.com/bonus948/nurseaceifn**](mometrix.com/bonus948/nurseaceifn)